Pediatric Coding Basics

An Introduction to Medical Coding

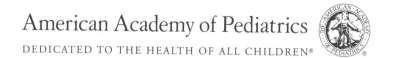

American Academy of Pediatrics
DEDICATED TO THE HEALTH OF ALL CHILDREN®

American Academy of Pediatrics Publishing Staff

Mary Lou White, *Chief Product and Services Officer/SVP, Membership, Marketing, and Publishing*
Mark Grimes, *Vice President, Publishing*
Mary Kelly, *Senior Editor, Professional/Clinical Publishing*
Jason Crase, *Senior Manager, Production and Editorial Services*
Leesa Levin-Doroba, *Production Manager, Practice Management*
Maryjo Reynolds, *Marketing Manager, Practice Publications*

Published by the American Academy of Pediatrics
345 Park Blvd
Itasca, IL 60143
Telephone: 630/626-6000
Facsimile: 847/434-8000
www.aap.org

The American Academy of Pediatrics is an organization of 67,000 primary care pediatricians, pediatric medical subspecialists, and pediatric surgical specialists dedicated to the health, safety, and well-being of infants, children, adolescents, and young adults.

While every effort has been made to ensure the accuracy of this publication, the American Academy of Pediatrics (AAP) does not guarantee that it is accurate, complete, or without error.

The recommendations in this publication do not indicate an exclusive course of treatment or serve as a standard of medical care. Variations, taking into account individual circumstances, may be appropriate. Vignettes are provided to illustrate correct coding applications and are not intended to offer advice on the practice of medicine.

Any websites, brand names, products, or manufacturers are mentioned for informational and identification purposes only and do not imply an endorsement by the American Academy of Pediatrics (AAP). The AAP is not responsible for the content of external resources. Information was current at the time of publication.

This publication has been developed by the American Academy of Pediatrics. The contributors are expert authorities in the field of pediatrics. No commercial involvement of any kind has been solicited or accepted in development of the content of this publication. Ms Arnold disclosed a consulting relationship with ThermoFisher Scientific. Dr Lago disclosed an employee relationship with Cotiviti, Inc. Dr Parsi disclosed an ownership and consulting relationship with The PEDS MD Company.

Special discounts are available for bulk purchases of this publication. Email Special Sales at aapsales@aap.org for more information.

Printed in the United States of America.

CPT® copyright 2019 American Medical Association (AMA). All rights reserved.

Fee schedules, relative value units, conversion factors, and/or related components are not assigned by the AMA, are not part of *CPT*, and the AMA is not recommending their use. The AMA does not directly or indirectly practice medicine or dispense medical services. The AMA assumes no liability for data contained or not contained herein.

CPT® is a registered trademark of the AMA.

11-128/0420   1 2 3 4 5 6 7 8 9 10

MA0968
ISBN: 978-1-61002-404-4
eBook: 978-1-61002-405-1

Cover and publication design by Wild Onion Design, Inc.

Library of Congress Control Number: 2020930105

Acknowledgments

The American Academy of Pediatrics would like to acknowledge the tireless work of the members of the Committee on Coding and Nomenclature. We especially thank the following members for their contributions to this publication:

Jeffrey F. Linzer Sr, MD, FAAP

Richard A. Molteni, MD, FAAP

Greg Barabell, MD, CPC, FAAP

Contents

Welcome and Overview

Welcome to *Pediatric Coding Basics: An Introduction to Medical Coding!* If you are ready to learn about coding for professional services in the practice of pediatric medicine, *Pediatric Coding Basics* is a great place to start. This introduction to the code sets and the reporting method used by physicians to bill health plans and other payers for services is a first step in learning to appropriately assign and report codes.

This book addresses gaps often seen by pediatricians and other health care professionals as they begin practicing and billing for their professional services. Too often pediatricians and other health care professionals were provided with paper or electronic lists from which they were to select codes without the benefit of

- Understanding where these codes come from
- How code selection affects payment for services
- Risks associated with incorrect code assignment

With that in mind, the American Academy of Pediatrics (AAP) and its Committee on Coding and Nomenclature developed this publication to provide background and basic information necessary to support appropriate code selection for specific conditions and services.

Pediatric Coding Basics begins with an overview of medical coding, followed by a more detailed review of the different types of codes commonly used in pediatrics. It then discusses how to effectively use the different types of codes together for billing purposes before exploring health plan policies and coding compliance. Each chapter includes Coding Challenge questions with the answers appearing in Appendix A. Appendix B is a glossary of commonly used acronyms and Appendix C includes a brief history of coding. Upon completion of this book, refer to Appendix D to learn how to take an online assessment and earn a Certificate of Completion from the AAP.

When you are ready to learn more about coding for pediatric services, we hope that you will take advantage of all the award-winning AAP coding products. These products empower pediatricians to code their work correctly with excellent explanations in addition to multiple helpful pediatric vignettes for general pediatricians as well as for subspecialists.

All *Current Procedural Terminology* (*CPT*®) and *International Classification of Diseases, 10th Revision, Clinical Modification* (*ICD-10-CM*) codes included in this publication are for educational purposes to understand the code sets. As of 2020 these codes are current; however, refer to the most current code-specific publication for up-to-date coding information.

Chapter 1

Introduction to Medical Coding

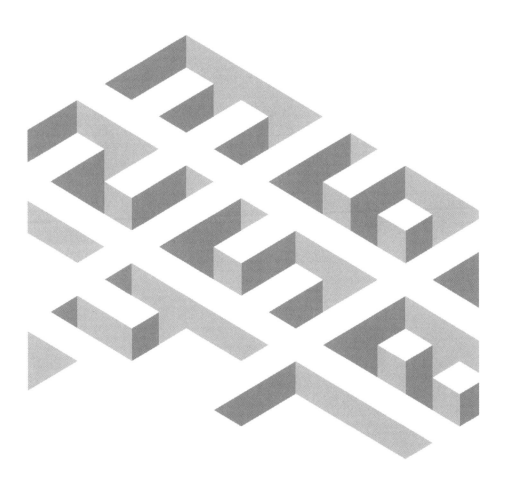

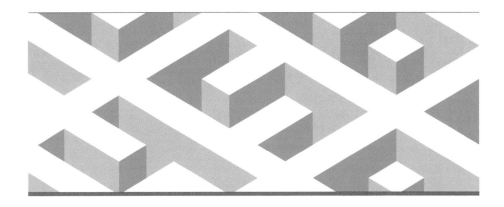

Introduction to Medical Coding

Medical coding is the translation of health information documented in a patient record to standardized codes. Codes can be included on health care claims and used for research, for population health management, and to inform injury prevention efforts. In this chapter, we will look at how pediatricians use codes with specific attention to use of codes to receive payment for services.

What Codes Do Pediatricians Use?

Pediatricians use 4 types of codes (**Table 1-1**) to create a picture of each patient encounter. Diagnosis codes (*International Classification of Diseases, 10th Revision, Clinical Modification* [*ICD-10-CM*]) and procedures codes (*Current Procedural Terminology* [*CPT*®] and Healthcare Common Procedure Coding System [HCPCS]), along with National Drug Codes (NDCs), are discussed in detail in chapters 2, 3, and 4.

Table 1-1. Code Sets Required by Health Insurance Portability and Accountability Act of 1996		
Code Set	**Used to Report**	**Examples**
International Classification of Diseases, 10th Revision, Clinical Modification (*ICD-10-CM*)	Diagnoses and other reasons for encounters, including status issues affecting care	**Z38.00** Single liveborn infant, delivered vaginally **J00** Acute nasopharyngitis (common cold)
Current Procedural Terminology (*CPT*®)[a]	• Most professional services • Vaccine and immune globulin products • Tracking performance measurement	**99238** Hospital discharge day management; 30 minutes or less **90680** Rotavirus vaccine, pentavalent (RV5), 3 dose schedule, live, for oral use
Healthcare Common Procedure Coding System (HCPCS)[b]	• Supplies • Medications • Services (when a *CPT* code does not describe the service as covered by health plan benefits)	**S0630** Removal of sutures; by a physician other than the physician who originally closed the wound **J0696** Rocephin per 250 mg
National Drug Code (NDC) (typically assigned by clinical staff)	• Specific prescription drugs • Vaccines • Insulin products • Dosages	**00006-4047-10** RotaTeq 2-mL single-dose tube, package of 10 **60574-4114-01** Synagis 0.5-mL in 1 vial, single dose

[a] Also known as Level I of the HCPCS code set.
[b] Refers to the Level II HCPCS codes maintained by the Centers for Medicare & Medicaid Services.

Why Pediatricians Use Codes

For the practicing pediatrician, most of the focus of coding is currently fee-for-service payment. A self-employed physician most directly sees the effect of correct coding, as practice revenue is largely dependent on reporting correct codes for procedures with supporting diagnosis codes. Many employment contracts tie physician pay to work relative value units (RVUs) assigned to each procedure code and to quality measurement that is largely dependent on complete documentation and accurate coding of conditions evaluated or managed at each encounter. **Box 1-1** includes more information about how these values are used in calculating payment for physician services.

Newer payment models may result in higher or lower payment based on the cost to provide care in relation to the expected health risks in a patient population. Diagnosis and procedure codes are used in determining risk and effectiveness of care.

All pediatricians are responsible for and affected by the quality of the documentation and coding of their services.

- Without accurate coding, payment may be delayed, denied, underpaid, or overpaid.
- Inaccurate coding can result in audits and recovery of amounts previously paid by health plans.
- Coding without an understanding of the official guidelines and instructions of each code set greatly increases the risk of investigation for abusive or fraudulent billing practices.

Additionally, all health claims include the pediatrician's certification that the information on the claim is accurate (**Figure 1-1**). Physicians do not actually have to sign each claim; rather, the signature field can state "Signature on File" and/or include a computer-generated signature.

Figure 1-1. 1500 Claim Form Certification

SIGNATURE OF PHYSICIAN OR SUPPLIER (MEDICARE, TRICARE, FECA AND BLACK LUNG)

In submitting this claim for payment from federal funds, I certify that: 1) the information on this form is true, accurate and complete; 2) I have familiarized myself with all applicable laws, regulations, and program instruction, which are available from the Medicare contractor; 3) I have provided or will provide sufficient information required to allow the government to make an informed eligibility and payment decision;... .

Box 1-1. More About Relative Value Units

Each code is assigned relative value units (RVUs) that are multiplied times a conversion factor (CF) to determine a health plan's payment.

- The relative value of each service is quantifiable and is based on the concept that there are 3 components of each service.

  > Physician work (approximately 50% of total RVUs)

  > Practice expense (approximately 44% of total RVUs)

  > Professional liability (approximately 4% of total RVUs)

- Payers multiply RVUs times a monetary CF or contracted fee schedule amount to determine allowed amounts (total payment from payer and patient) for physician services.

  > The Medicare CF was $36.0896 in 2020.

  > Medicare uses geographic practice cost indexes (GPCIs) to adjust RVUs based on the cost of practicing in specific localities (eg, Baltimore, MD, versus rest of Maryland). Other payers may or may not use the same methodology.

  > Individual health plans may offer different conversion factors. These are typically specified in network participation contracts.

- Relative value units are lower in facility settings (eg, hospital) than in non-facility settings (eg, physician office) because the practice expense is lower for facility-based professional services (ie, the facility pays and is paid for overhead expenses).

Example

A health plan uses the 2020 Medicare Physician Fee Schedule (MPFS) as a basis for payment with a CF of $38 per RVU. A physician submits established patient preventive medicine visit code **99392** to the plan. The total Medicare non-facility RVUs (3.01) assigned to code **99392** are multiplied by the $38 CF to determine the allowed amount for the service.

(Total Medicare RVUs) × (payer CF) = allowed amount

(3.01) × ($38) = $114.38

Actual payment may vary based on the patient's out-of-pocket obligation. The total non-facility RVUs are a combination of RVUs for physician work (1.50), non-facility practice expense (1.40), and professional liability (0.11).

- Private health plans often use the MPFS as the basis of their fee schedules for paying physicians. However, plans may use MPFS from prior years. Be aware when signing contracts with health plans.

Work RVUs are often used by employers to measure physician productivity and may be directly used in determining salaries. Work RVUs are not affected by the site of service (facility or non-facility).

Example

A pediatrician receives credit for 1.50 work RVUs when providing a preventive medicine service to an established patient. The practice is paid based on the 3.01 total RVUs (or 2.19 total RVUs in a facility setting) to cover the costs associated with operating the clinic (eg, building, clinical and clerical staff, supplies).

Getting Paid

The Health Insurance Portability and Accountability Act of 1996 (HIPAA) mandated specific claim forms (electronic and paper) and codes for reporting medical services. HIPAA regulations allow use of

- Electronic 837 Health Care Claim: Professionals or 1500 paper claim form (discussed more later in this chapter)
- *Current Procedural Terminology* or HCPCS codes for services (payers are not required to comply with *CPT* instructions)
- The current version of the US clinical modification of the *International Classification of Diseases* (currently *ICD-10-CM*), including official guidelines for reporting

Standardization increased use of electronic data to not only file claims but verify patient health plan eligibility and plan benefits, download reports of claims accepted or rejected by a payer, and receive electronic reports of claims paid or denied.

Documentation and Coding

Codes are assigned based only on what is documented in the patient record. For this reason, much of coding education is focused on the documentation necessary to support code assignment.

No code shall be assigned without supporting documentation.

The 1995 and 1997 *Documentation Guidelines for Evaluation and Management Services* include the following section called "General Principles of Medical Record Documentation":

1. The medical record should be complete and legible.

2. The documentation of each patient encounter should include

   > Reason for the encounter and relevant history, physical examination findings, and prior diagnostic test results

   > Assessment, clinical impression, or diagnosis

   > Plan for care

   > Date and legible identity of the observer

3. If not documented, the rationale for ordering diagnostic and other ancillary services should be easily inferred.

4. Past and present diagnoses should be accessible to the treating and/or consulting physician.

5. Appropriate health risk factors should be identified.

6. The patient's progress, response to and changes in treatment, and revision of diagnosis should be documented.

7. The *CPT* and *ICD-10-CM* codes reported on the health insurance claim form or billing statement should be supported by the documentation in the medical record.

Additionally, documentation should reflect all of a pediatrician's work but not overstate the service provided (eg, checklists should not indicate examinations of body areas not actually examined at an encounter).

Never alter a medical record entry by deleting text or add to completed documentation without noting the addendum and including your signature and the current date.

Documentation is not complete if it is not authenticated.

Documentation is not complete if it is not authenticated by the pediatrician and/or clinical staff member who performed and documented each service. All documentation should be signed (written or electronic) and dated. Auditors routinely deny claims when supporting documentation is not authenticated.

Complete, timely, and accurate documentation is mostly important for ongoing patient care. However, because of the link between documentation and payment for services provided, pediatricians must hold to a high standard of integrity for medical record documentation. Ideally, each pediatric practice will develop and maintain documentation standards and require all clinical staff to conform to these standards.

Failure to accurately document services and assign codes based on the services performed and supported by the documentation can lead to compliance risks, including increased chance of audit and demands for refund by health plans.

Code Assignment

Coding often involves several people with differing roles.

- Pediatricians and other health care professionals document services and diagnoses/reasons for services and often select codes in an electronic health record or from lists of commonly used codes (often referred to as *superbills* [**Figure 1-2**]).

- Professional certified coders may select codes based on documentation or may review codes selected by pediatricians for accuracy and completeness prior to billing.

- Practice administrators and technology support staff often select and/or create tools for use by physicians and coders (eg, electronic health record documentation templates and code selection lists).

- Compliance teams typically include physicians and/or coding professionals who take responsibility for maintaining documentation standards and compliant coding in a practice or facility through education, internal chart reviews, and review of compliance with practice policies and procedures.

Tips for better documentation and code selection are included in the discussion of each code set. See Chapter 6 for an overview of compliance topics such as medical necessity, global periods, and coding edits used in claims adjudication.

Figure 1-2. American Academy of Pediatrics Superbill

Pediatric Office Superbill 2020

NEW	OFFICE VISITS	EST
-	Clinical staff-5 min	99211
99201	Office/OP-10 min	99212
-	Office/OP-15 min	99213
99202	Office/OP-20 min	-
-	Office/OP-25 min	99214
99203	Office/OP-30 min	-
-	Office/OP-40 min	99215
99204	Office/OP-45 min	-
99205	Office/OP-60 min	-

OFFICE/OUTPATIENT CONSULTATIONS	
99241	Office consultation-15 min
99242	Office consultation-30 min
99243	Office consultation-40 min
99244	Office consultation-60 min
99245	Office consultation-80 min

PROLONGED SERVICES	
+99354	Office/OP dir contact-1st h
+99355	Office/OP dir contact addl-30 min No.___
99358	Before/after dir care-1st h
+99359	Before/after dir care addl-30 min No.___
+99415	Clinical staff-1st h
+99416	Clinical staff addl-30 min No.___

NEW	PREVENTIVE MEDICINE	EST
99381	<1 y	99391
99382	1-4 y	99392
99383	5-11 y	99393
99384	12-17 y	99394
99385	18-39 y	99395

PREVENTIVE MEDICINE COUNSELING	
99401	15 min
99402	30 min
99403	45 min
99404	60 min
99406	Smoking cessation-3-10 min
99407	Smoking cessation->10 min
99408	AUDIT/DAST w/ SBI-15-30 min
99409	AUDIT/DAST w/ SBI->30 min

HOURLY CRITICAL CARE	
99291	Critical care-1st h
+99292	Critical care-addl 30 min

ADD-ON SERVICES	
99050	Medical services after hours
99051	Medical services eve/wkend/holiday
99058	Office emerg care
99060	Out of office emerg medical service

IMMUNIZATION ADMINISTRATION	
90460	IA <19 y any rte 1st/only comp No.___
+90461	IA <19 y any rte addl comp No.___
90471	IA 1st vaccine IM/SQ
+90472	IA each addl vaccine IM/SC No.___
90473	IA intransl/oral 1st vaccine
+90474	IA intransl/oral each addl vaccine No.___

IMMUNIZATIONS (CONTINUED)	
90672	Flu, quadrivalent, live, intransl
90674	Flu, quadrivalent, cell cultured, no preserv or antibiotic, 0.5 mL dose, IM
90756	Flu, quadrivalent, cell cultured, no antibiotic, 0.5 mL dose, IM
90685	Flu, no preserv, quadrivalent, 0.25 mL dose, IM
90686	Flu, no preserv, quadrivalent, 0.5 mL dose, IM
90687	Flu, quadrivalent, 0.25 mL dose, IM
90688	Flu, quadrivalent, 0.5 mL dose, IM
90656	Flu, no preserv, trivalent, 0.5 mL dose, IM
90658	Flu, trivalent, 0.5 mL dose, IM
90633	Hep A, 2 dose, IM
90743	Hep B, adol, 2 dose, IM
90744	Hep B, ped/adol, 3 dose, IM
90647	Hib, PRP-OMP, 3 dose, IM
90648	Hib, PRP-T, 4 dose, IM
90651	HPV, nonvalent, 2 or 3 dose, IM
90713	IPV, SQ or IM
90620	Meningococcal, serogroup B (MenB-4C), 2 dose, IM
90621	Meningococcal, serogroup B (MenB-FHbp), 2 or 3 dose, IM
90734	Meningococcal conj, quadrivalent, IM
90707	MMR, SQ
90710	MMRV, SQ
90670	Pneumococcal, 13 valent, IM
90732	Pneumococcal polysac, 23 valent, ≥2y, SQ or IM
90680	Rotavirus, 3 dose, oral
90681	Rotavirus, 2 dose, oral
90715	Tdap, ≥7 y, IM
90716	Varicella (chickenpox), SQ
Other	

SURGICAL PROCEDURES	
10060	Incision & drainage, abscess
10120	Incision & removal FB skin, simple
120__	Simple repair loc ___ size ___
16000	Initial treatment of burn(s), local
16020	Dress/debride p-thick burn(s), small (<5% TBSA)
17110	Destruct benign lesion 1-14
17111	Destruct benign lesion ≥15
17250	Chemical cautery tissue
24640	Treat elbow disl (nursemaid elbow)
28190	Removal FB foot, SQ
30300	Removal FB intransl
30901	Control nosebleed
51701	Insert bladder catheter
65205	Removal FB from eye
69200	Removal FB external auditory canal
69209	Removal impacted earwax-irrigation/lavage, ___ bilat
69210	Removal impacted earwax, ___ bilat

OTHER PROCEDURES	
92551	Screen test pure tone, air only
92552	Pure tone, threshold, air only
92567	Tympanometry

OTHER PROCEDURES (CONTINUED)	
94760	Noninvasive ear/pulse ox single
96110	Developmental screen No.___
96127	Emotional/behavioral assmt No.___
No.	IV infusion hydration-initial 31 min-1 h
+96361	IV infusion hydration-each addl h
99173	Vision screen, acuity
99174	Instrument-based ocular screen, remote analysis
99177	Instrument-based ocular screen, w/ on-site analysis
99188	Application topical fluoride varnish
96160	Health risk assmt, patient No.___
96161	Health risk assmt, caregiver No.___
Other	

INJECTIONS	
95115	Allergy inj, 1
95117	Allergy inj, >1
96372	Therapeutic proph/dx inj SQ/IM

LABORATORY	
81000	Urinalysis nonauto w/ scope
81002	Urinalysis nonauto w/o scope
82272	Blood occult peroxidase actv qual feces, 1-3 specimen
82948	Glucose blood reagent strip
82962	Glucose blood
85018	Blood count hemoglobin
86308	Heterophile antibodies screen
86580	Skin test, TB, intradermal
87070	Culture, other specimen, aerobic
87086	Urine culture/colony count
87430	Strep A, enzyme immunoassay
87804	Influenza, rapid A ___ B ___
87880	Strep A, rapid
36405	Venipuncture, <3 y, phys/qhp skill, scalp vein
36406	Venipuncture, <3 y, phys/qhp skill, other vein
36410	Venipuncture, ≥3 y, phys/qhp skill
36415	Collection venous blood venipuncture
36416	Collection capillary blood specimen
99000	Specimen handling, office-lab
Other	

INJECTED MEDICATIONS	
J1200	Benadryl up to 50 mg
J0558	Bicillin C-R 100,000 units No.___
J0561	Bicillin L-A 100,000 units No.___
J1100	Decadron 1 mg No.___
J0171	Epinephrine 0.1 mg
J2550	Phenergan up to 50 mg
J0696	Rocephin per 250 mg No.___
90378	RSV IM use, per 50 mg (Synagis) No.___

OTHER MEDICATIONS	
J7611	Albuterol, inhal, concentrated, 1 mg
J7612	Levalbuterol, inhal, concentrated, 0.5 mg
J7613	Albuterol, inhal, unit, 1 mg

DIAGNOSIS	
R10.84	Abdominal pain, generalized
R10.3-	Abdominal pain, lower: 0 unspec; 1 RLQ; 2 LLO; 3 periumbilical
R10.1-	Abdominal pain, upper: 0 unspec; 1 RUQ; 2 LUQ; 3 epigastric
H93.29-	Abnormal auditory perceptions: 1 rt; 2 lt; 3 bilat
R73.09	Abnormal glucose level
R25.0	Abnormal head movements
P09	Abnormal neonatal screen
R76.11	Abnormal TB test results
By site*	Abrasion, site ___
L02.-	Abscess, cutaneous/carbuncle/furuncle site ___ infectious ___ noninfectious
L70.-	Acne: 0 vulgaris; 1 conglobata; 2 varioliformis; 4 infantile; 8 other; 9 unspec
F90.0	ADD
F90.1	ADHD
N89.5	Adhesions, vaginal
F43.20	Adjustment disorder, unspec
F10.10	Alcohol abuse, uncomplicated
F10.20	Alcohol dependence, uncomplicated
J30.-	Allergic rhinitis d/t: 1 pollen (hay fever); 2 other (seasonal); 5 food; 9 unspec
J30.8-	Allergic rhinitis d/t: 1 animal (cat/dog); 9 other
H53.04-	Amblyopia, suspect: 1 rt; 2 lt; 3 bilat
N91.-	Amenorrhea: 0 primary; 1 secondary; 2 unspec
D50.9	Anemia, iron deficiency, unspec
R63.0	Anorexia (loss of appetite)
F41.1	Anxiety disorder, generalized
F41.9	Anxiety disorder, unspec
Q23.0	Aortic valve stenosis, congenital
R06.81	Apnea, child
P28.-	Apnea, NB: 3 sleep; 4 other (pre-maturity)
G47.30	Apnea, sleep, unspec
J45.991	Asthma, cough variant
J45.2-	Asthma, mild intermittent:
J45.3-	Asthma, mild persistent:
J45.4-	Asthma, moderate persistent:
J45.5-	Asthma, severe persistent: 0 uncomplicated; 1 w/ (acute) exacerbation; 2 w/ status asthmaticus
Q21.1	Atrial septal defect, congenital
Q21.2	Atrioventricular septal defect
F84.0	Autism
R78.81	Bacteremia
P07.0-	Birth weight, extreme low ___ g
P07.1-	Birth weight, low ___ g
Z68.51	BMI, ped, <5th percentile for age
Z68.52	5th-<85th percentile for age
Z68.53	85th-<95th percentile for age
Z68.54	≥95th percentile for age
P83.4	Breast engorgement, NB
J21.0	Bronchiolitis, acute, d/t RSV
J21.9	Bronchiolitis, acute, unspec organism
J98.01	Bronchospasm, acute
J45.990	Bronchospasm, exercise induced

Coding Keys

- **Medical coding in a nutshell:** Medical coding is the translation of health information documented in a patient record to standardized codes.

- **There are 4 code sets used by pediatricians.**

  > *International Classification of Diseases, 10th Revision, Clinical Modification* (*ICD-10-CM*)

  > Current Procedural Technology (*CPT*)

  > Healthcare Common Procedure Coding System (HCPCS)

  > National Drug Code (NDC)

- **Relative value units (RVUs) explained:** RVUs are figures assigned to procedure codes that are multiplied by a conversion factor (CF) to determine a health plan's payment to a physician. They are based on the concept that there are 3 components of each service: physician work, practice expense, and professional liability.

- **Inaccurate coding can cause big problems.** Inaccurate coding can lead to payments being delayed, denied, underpaid, or overpaid. It can also lead to audits and recovery of amounts previously paid by health plans. Inaccurate coding also greatly increases the risk of investigation of potentially abusive or fraudulent billing practices.

- **Health Insurance Portability and Accountability Act of 1996 (HIPAA) mandates require specific claim forms and codes for reporting medical services.**

  > Electronic 837 Health Care Claim: Professionals or 1500 paper claim form

  > *CPT* or HCPCS codes for services

  > The current version of the US clinical modification of the *International Classification of Diseases* (currently *ICD-10-CM*), including official guidelines for reporting

- **There are 7 general principles of medical record documentation.**

  1. The medical record should be complete and legible.

  2. The documentation of each patient encounter should include the reason for the encounter and relevant history, physical examination findings, and prior diagnostic test results; assessment, clinical impression, or diagnosis; plan for care; and date and legible identity of the observer.

  3. If not documented, the rationale for ordering diagnostic and other ancillary services should be easily inferred.

  4. Past and present diagnoses should be accessible to the treating and/or consulting physician.

  5. Appropriate health risk factors should be identified.

  6. The patient's progress, response to and changes in treatment, and revision of diagnosis should be documented.

  7. The *CPT* and *ICD-10-CM* codes reported on the health insurance claim form or billing statement should be supported by the documentation in the medical record.

- **Multiple individuals play roles in the coding process.**
  - > **Pediatricians and other health care professionals** document services and diagnoses/reasons for services and often select codes in electronic health records (EHRs) or on superbills.
  - > **Professional certified coders** select codes based on documentation or may review codes selected by pediatricians for accuracy and completeness.
  - > **Practice administrators and technology support staff** select and/or create tools to be used by physicians and coders.
  - > **Compliance teams** maintain documentation standards and compliant coding through education, internal chart reviews, and review of compliance with practice policies and procedures.

Resources

American Academy of Pediatrics

- *AAP Pediatric Coding Newsletter*™ (http://coding.aap.org)
- Coding Hotline (www.aap.org/en-us/Pages/cu/Coding-Hotline-Request.aspx)
- Coding Webinars (www.aap.org/en-us/professional-resources/practice-transformation/getting-paid/Coding-at-the-AAP/Pages/AAP-Coding-Webinars.aspx)
- *Pediatric Office Superbill* (https://shop.aap.org)

Current Procedural Terminology®

- American Academy of Pediatrics *Coding for Pediatrics* (www.aap.org/cfp)
- American Medical Association *CPT* general information (www.ama-assn.org/practice-management/cpt-current-procedural-terminology)

Documentation

- 1995 and 1997 *Documentation Guidelines for Evaluation and Management Services* (www.aap.org/cfp)
- American Academy of Pediatrics Pediatric Visit Documentation Forms for office or outpatient visits (http://shop.aap.org)

International Classification of Diseases, 10th Revision, Clinical Modification Code Files and Guidelines

- American Academy of Pediatrics *Pediatric ICD-10-CM: A Manual for Provider-Based Coding* (https://shop.aap.org)
- National Center for Health Statistics *ICD-10-CM* (www.cdc.gov/nchs/icd/icd10cm.htm)

National Drug Codes

- US Food and Drug Administration National Drug Code Directory (www.fda.gov/drugs/informationondrugs/ucm142438.htm)

Payment/Relative Value Units

- "2020 RBRVS: What Is It and How Does It Affect Pediatrics?" (https://www.aap.org/en-us/professional-resources/practice-transformation/getting-paid/Coding-at-the-AAP/Pages/Code-Valuation-and-PaymentRBRVS.aspx; access code AAPCFP25)
- "Pediatric Application of Coding and Valuation Systems" (https://pediatrics.aappublications.org/content/144/4/e20192496)
- "Understanding the RUC Survey Instrument: Physician Services" video (www.youtube.com/watch?v=nu5unDX8Vls)

- American Academy of Pediatrics Code Valuation and Payment RBRVS (https://www.aap.org/en-us/professional-resources/practice-transformation/getting-paid/Coding-at-the-AAP/Pages/Code-Valuation-and-PaymentRBRVS.aspx)

- American Academy of Pediatrics Managed Care Contracting (www.aap.org/en-us/professional-resources/practice-transformation/getting-paid/Pages/managed-care-contracting.aspx)

- American Academy of Pediatrics Resources for Payment (www.aap.org/en-us/professional-resources/practice-transformation/getting-paid/Pages/resources-for-payment.aspx)

Coding Challenge

(Answers may be found in Appendix A.)

1. How many Health Insurance Portability and Accountability Act of 1996 (HIPAA)-designated code sets can be used in reporting pediatric professional services?

    a. 2

    b. 3

    c. 4

    d. 5

2. The rationale for ordering diagnostic and other ancillary services should be what?

    a. Included on the claim form

    b. Documented

    c. Easily inferred

    d. b and c

3. Which of the following is mandated by HIPAA?

    a. Everyone must have health insurance.

    b. Codes for reporting medical services

    c. Specific claim forms (electronic and paper)

    d. b and c

4. Who certifies the correctness of the information on each claim submitted for payment?

    a. The billing staff who prepare claims for submission

    b. The pediatrician or other provider of service

    c. The patient

    d. A practice manager or administrator

Chapter 2

Diagnosis Coding

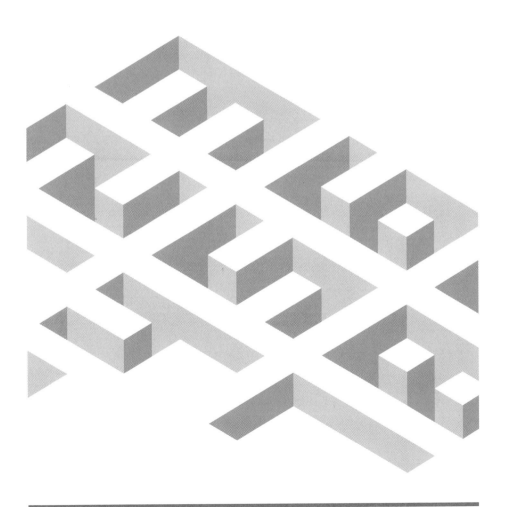

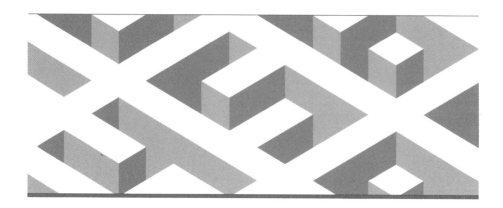

Diagnoses

Every encounter should begin with documentation of the patient's or caregiver's reason for the encounter. This reason, or *chief complaint*, leads to services and documentation of diagnoses (eg, well child with no abnormal findings, allergic rhinitis). Sometimes, the chief complaint is also the final diagnosis at the end of the encounter (eg, a problem that requires further workup to determine a diagnosis). Diagnosis codes are used to report the reasons that services were provided. A diagnosis should always be supported by documentation in the medical record for that encounter.

International Classification of Diseases, 10th Revision, Clinical Modification (*ICD-10-CM*) was adopted by the United States on October 1, 2015, for reporting diagnoses on health care claims. Recently, the World Health Organization (WHO) has approved *International Classification of Diseases, 11th Revision* (*ICD-11*), which will eventually be modified for use in the United States. The *ICD-11* has been developed specifically for use in electronic format. The US transition from *ICD-10-CM* to *ICD-11*-CM will happen only after appropriate regulatory notices from the Centers for Medicare & Medicaid Services. This is a lengthy process subject to industry readiness and acceptance.

International Classification of Diseases, 10th Revision, Clinical Modification (*ICD-10-CM*)

Diagnosis coding with *ICD-10-CM* is important to pediatricians because codes provide data to support public health efforts and resource utilization, as well as payment. **Table 2-1** provides a quick reference to the diagnosis code set, its uses, and when it is effective.

Table 2-1. *International Classification of Diseases, 10th Revision, Clinical Modification* (*ICD-10-CM*)	
Used to Report	**Effective Date**
Diagnoses and other reasons for encounters, including status issues affecting care	Annually, October 1 April 1 for emerging issues

Diagnosis codes are assigned to diagnoses and reasons for encounters as documented in the patient record and not in place of a specific statement of the pediatrician's assessment of the patient's condition. If a definitive diagnosis has not been established by the end of the encounter, it is appropriate to report codes for sign(s) and/or symptom(s) in lieu of a definitive diagnosis.

Example

A diagnosis of cough and chest discomfort, probable gastroesophageal reflux, is reported with codes R05 (cough) and R07.89 (other chest pain). *ICD-10-CM* codes alone do not provide sufficient detail for clinical follow-up but do provide sufficient detail for payment purposes.

An *ICD-10-CM* manual is composed of multiple sections (**Figure 2-1**).

Figure 2-1. Sections Within the *International Classification of Diseases, 10th Revision, Clinical Modification (ICD-10-CM)* Manual

Official Guidelines for Coding and Reporting

ICD-10-CM Official Guidelines for Coding and Reporting
FY 2020
(October 1, 2019 - September 30, 2020)

Narrative changes appear in bold text
Items <u>underlined</u> have been moved within the guidelines since the FY 2019 version
Italics are used to indicate revisions to heading changes

The Centers for Medicare and Medicaid Services (CMS) and the National Center for Health Statistics (NCHS), two departments within the U.S. Federal Government's Department of Health and Human Services (DHHS) provide the following guidelines for coding and reporting using the International Classification of Diseases, 10th Revision, Clinical Modification (ICD-10-CM). These guidelines should be used as a companion document to the official version of the ICD-10-CM as published on the NCHS website. The ICD-10-CM is a morbidity classification published

Alphabetic Index to Diseases and Injuries

ICD-10-CM INDEX TO DISEASES and INJURIES

A

Aarskog's syndrome Q87.19
Abandonment -*see* Maltreatment
Abasia (-astasia) (hysterical) F44.4
Abderhalden-Kaufmann-Lignac syndrome (cystinosis) E72.04
Abdomen, abdominal -*see also* condition
- acute R10.0
- angina K55.1
- muscle deficiency syndrome Q79.4
Abdominalgia -*see* Pain, abdominal
Abduction contracture, hip or other joint -*see* Contraction, joint
Aberrant (congenital) -*see also* Malposition, congenital
- adrenal gland Q89.1
- artery (peripheral) Q27.8
- - basilar NEC Q28.1
- - cerebral Q28.3

Table of Drugs and Chemicals

ICD-10-CM TABLE of DRUGS and CHEMICALS

Substance	Poisoning Accidental (unintentional)	Poisoning Intentional self-harm	Poisoning Assault	Poisoning Undetermined	Adverse effect	Underdosing
1-propanol	T51.3X1	T51.3X2	T51.3X3	T51.3X4	--	--
2-propanol	T51.2X1	T51.2X2	T51.2X3	T51.2X4	--	--
2,4-D (dichlorophen-oxyacetic acid)	T60.3X1	T60.3X2	T60.3X3	T60.3X4	--	--
2,4-toluene diisocyanate	T65.0X1	T65.0X2	T65.0X3	T65.0X4	--	--
2,4,5-T (trichloro-phenoxyacetic acid)	T60.1X1	T60.1X2	T60.1X3	T60.1X4	--	--
3,4-methylenedioxymethamphetamine	T43.641	T43.642	T43.643	T43.644	--	--
14-hydroxydihydro-morphinone	T40.2X1	T40.2X2	T40.2X3	T40.2X4	T40.2X5	T40.2X6

ICD-10-CM TABLE of NEOPLASMS

The list below gives the code numbers for neoplasms by anatomical site. For each site there are six possible code numbers according to whether the neoplasm in question is malignant, benign, in situ, of uncertain behavior, or of unspecified nature. The description of the neoplasm will often indicate which of the six columns is appropriate; e.g., malignant melanoma of skin, benign fibroadenoma of breast, carcinoma in situ of cervix uteri.

Codes listed with a dash (-) following the code have a required additional character for laterality. The Tabular must be reviewed for the complete code.

Neoplasm	Malignant Primary	Malignant Secondary	Ca in situ	Benign	Uncertain Behavior	Unspecified Behavior
Neoplasm, neoplastic	C80.1	C79.9	D09.9	D36.9	D48.9	D49.9
- abdomen, abdominal	C76.2	C79.8-	D09.8	D36.7	D48.7	D49.89
- - cavity	C76.2	C79.8-	D09.8	D36.7	D48.7	D49.89
- - organ	C76.2	C79.8-	D09.8	D36.7	D48.7	D49.89
- - viscera	C76.2	C79.8-	D09.8	D36.7	D48.7	D49.89
- - wall -*see also Neoplasm, abdomen, wall, skin*	C44.509	C79.2-	D04.5	D23.5	D48.5	D49.2
- - - connective tissue	C49.4	C79.8-	-	D21.4	D48.1	D49.2
- - - skin	C44.509	-	-	-	-	-
- - - - basal cell carcinoma	C44.519	-	-	-	-	-
- - cavity	C76.2	C79.8-	D09.8	D36.7	D48.7	D49.89

ICD-10-CM External Cause of Injuries Index

A

Abandonment (causing exposure to weather conditions) (with intent to injure or kill) NEC X58
Abuse (adult) (child) (mental) (physical) (sexual) X58
Accident (to) X58
- aircraft (in transit) (powered) -*see also* Accident, transport, aircraft
- - due to, caused by cataclysm -*see* Forces of nature, by type
- animal-rider -*see* Accident, transport, animal-rider
- animal-drawn vehicle -*see* Accident, transport, animal-drawn vehicle occupant
- automobile -*see* Accident, transport, car occupant
- bare foot water skiier V94.4
- boat, boating -*see also* Accident, watercraft

External Causes of Injury

ICD-10-CM includes codes to specify the cause of injuries. Although not required in all settings, these help health plans identify claims that are covered by the plan or that may be payable by other sources, such as automobile insurance.

ICD-10-CM TABULAR LIST of DISEASES and INJURIES

Table of Contents

Manuals are available in print or electronic format (typically a software application). Downloadable files of the entire *ICD-10-CM* code set and guidelines are available without charge from the National Center for Health Statistics at www.cdc.gov/nchs/icd/icd10cm. htm.

- The tabular and index instructions take precedence over guidelines.
- Always start with the alphabetic indexes and follow instructions there to locate the appropriate code in the tabular list.
- Never select a code from the index alone because you may miss critical tabular guidance.
- Unlike *Current Procedural Terminology* (*CPT®*), the *ICD-10-CM* guidelines, tabular list, and alphabetic index must be followed per Health Insurance Portability and Accountability Act of 1996 (HIPAA) regulation.
- Inpatient *ICD-10-CM* guidelines are only applicable when assigning codes for the facility setting.

ICD-10-CM Guidelines

The guidelines are based on the coding and sequencing instructions in the tabular list and alphabetic index of *ICD-10-CM* but provide additional instruction. Sections I and IV of the guidelines apply when reporting services of health care professionals. HIPAA requires all covered entities (nearly all physicians and health plans) to adhere to *ICD-10-CM* guidelines when using *ICD-10-CM* codes for health care transactions (ie, prior authorizations, payment).

Table 2-2 provides some *ICD-10-CM* guideline tips that are most relevant to pediatric coding for conditions and reasons for encounters.

ICD-10-CM Tips

Chapters of the Tabular List of *ICD-10-CM*

1. Certain infectious and parasitic diseases (**A00–B99**)
2. Neoplasms (**C00–D49**)
3. Diseases of the blood and blood-forming organs and certain disorders involving the immune mechanism (**D50–D89**)
4. Endocrine, nutritional and metabolic diseases (**E00–E89**)
5. Mental, behavioral and neurodevelopmental disorders (**F01–F99**)
6. Diseases of the nervous system (**G00–G99**)
7. Diseases of the eye and adnexa (**H00–H59**)
8. Diseases of the ear and mastoid process (**H60–H95**)
9. Diseases of the circulatory system (**I00–I99**)
10. Diseases of the respiratory system (**J00–J99**)
11. Diseases of the digestive system (**K00–K95**)

12. Diseases of the skin and subcutaneous tissue (**L00–L99**)

13. Diseases of the musculoskeletal system and connective tissue (**M00–M99**)

14. Diseases of the genitourinary system (**N00–N99**)

15. Pregnancy, childbirth and the puerperium (**O00–O9A**)

    Reported only on mother's claims

16. Certain conditions originating in the perinatal period (**P00–P96**)

    Reported for any condition originating in the first 28 days after birth (day of birth is day 0) as long as the condition continues to exist and affect care

17. Congenital malformations, deformations and chromosomal abnormalities (**Q00–Q99**)

    Reported as long as condition remains and affects care. History of corrected congenital conditions may be reported with codes from Chapter 21, when applicable.

18. Symptoms, signs and abnormal clinical and laboratory findings, not elsewhere classified (**R00–R99**)

    Reported when not routinely associated with a diagnosed condition or in the absence of a diagnosis

19. Injury, poisoning and certain other consequences of external causes (**S00–T88**)

    - Seventh characters are typically required, most commonly
        > **A** (initial encounter [active treatment/management])
        > **D** (subsequent encounter [healing phase])
        > **S** (sequela [late effect of an injury such as scarring])
    - Always reference the tabular list for applicable seventh characters.

20. External causes of morbidity (**V00–Y99**)

    - Reporting is optional except when required by state regulations.
    - Seventh characters apply to codes **V00–Y38** (**A**, **D**, or **S**).
    - Codes from this section indicate the nature of the condition and are used as secondary codes.

21. Factors influencing health status and contact with health services (**Z00–Z99**)

    - Categories **Z00–Z99** are provided for occasions when circumstances other than a disease, injury, or external cause classifiable to categories **A00–Y89** are recorded as diagnoses or problems. This can arise in 2 main ways.
        > Encounters for health services for some specific purpose, such as evaluation after a motor vehicle crash with no signs or symptoms of injury, to receive prophylactic vaccination (immunization), or to discuss a problem which, in itself, is not a disease or injury
        > When some circumstance or problem is present which influences the person's health status but is not, in itself, a current illness or injury

22. Codes for special purposes (**U00–U85**)

- New chapter added April 1, 2020. Codes **U00–U49** are used by WHO for the provisional assignment of new diseases of uncertain etiology.

  > Only one code, **U07.0**, for vaping-related disorders, exists at the time of publication. Other codes will be added as needed.

Table 2-2. *ICD-10-CM* Guideline Tips	
Here are 2020 *ICD-10-CM* guidelines for a selection of topics listed with the section numbers where each can be found (eg, section I, subsection B, #5 is listed as §I.B.5). See current guidelines for full information.	
Code Assignment and Clinical Criteria	**§I.A.19** The assignment of a diagnosis code is based on the provider's diagnostic statement that the condition exists. The provider's statement that the patient has a particular condition is sufficient. Code assignment is not based on clinical criteria used by the provider to establish the diagnosis.
Locating Codes	**§I.B.1** To select a code in the classification that corresponds to a diagnosis or reason for visit documented in a medical record, first locate the term in the Alphabetic Index, and then verify the code in the Tabular List. Read and be guided by instructional notations that appear in both the Alphabetic Index and the Tabular List.
Signs and Symptoms	**§I.B.5** Signs and symptoms that are associated routinely with a disease process should not be assigned as additional codes, unless otherwise instructed by the classification. **§I.B.6** Additional signs and symptoms that may not be associated routinely with a disease process should be coded when present.
Unspecified Codes	**§I.B.18** When sufficient clinical information isn't known or available about a particular health condition to assign a more specific code, it is acceptable to report the appropriate "unspecified" code (eg, J18.9 [pneumonia, unspecified organism] is reported for pneumonia diagnosed without identification of the specific type). Unspecified codes should be reported when they are the codes that most accurately reflect what is known about the patient's condition at the time of that particular encounter.
"With" in a Code Title, Alphabetic Index, or Tabular List	**§I.A.15** • The word "with" in the Alphabetic Index is sequenced immediately following the main term, not in alphabetical order. • The word "with" or "in" should be interpreted to mean "associated with" or "due to" when it appears in a code title, the Alphabetic Index (either under a main term or sub-term), or an instructional note in the Tabular List.

Abbreviation: *ICD-10-CM, International Classification of Diseases, 10th Revision, Clinical Modification.*

> In *ICD-10-CM*, a code is a complete set of alphanumeric characters for which there are no further subdivisions.

Code Structure

ICD-10-CM codes are 3 to 7 characters long. The pattern is **XXX.XXXX**.

The first character of each code is a letter ranging from A to Z.

Although typically illustrated in capital letters, the alphabetic characters are not case sensitive.

- The second through seventh characters may be letters or numbers. For codes that extend beyond 3 characters, the first 3 characters are found to the left of a decimal, with the remaining characters to the right.

- Fourth through sixth characters indicate etiology, severity, site, manifestation(s) of an underlying etiology, or intent.

- When required, a seventh character adds information such as the episode of care or status of fracture healing.

> **Indication of Additionally Required Characters**
>
> When an incomplete code is referenced, the need for additional characters is typically indicated by a dash (-).
>
> For example, **J06.-** indicates that it is necessary to see an *International Classification of Diseases, 10th Revision, Clinical Modification* reference to select a complete code. Options for complete codes are
>
> **J06.0** Acute laryngopharyngitis
>
> **J06.9** Acute upper respiratory infection unspecified

  > The tabular list advises when a seventh character is required.

  > Seventh characters must be placed in the seventh place in a code. Letter **X** is used as a placeholder for fourth through sixth characters when necessary (eg, **T16.1XXA**, foreign body in right ear, initial encounter).

Examples of complete codes are illustrated in **Table 2-3**.

Code Selection

The *ICD-10-CM* coding manual instructs that code selection begins in the alphabetic index.

Example

You diagnose a child with influenza with cough and sore throat. You also document that the child is exposed to tobacco smoke frequently in the home.

Table 2-3. Examples of *ICD-10-CM* Codes	
J00	Acute nasopharyngitis [common cold]
J02.0	Streptococcal pharyngitis
J03.00 J03.01	Acute streptococcal tonsillitis, unspecified Acute recurrent streptococcal tonsillitis
H60.331 H60.332 H60.333	Swimmer's ear, right ear Swimmer's ear, left ear Swimmer's ear, bilateral
S40.621A S40.621D S40.621S	Insect bite (nonvenomous) of right shoulder, initial encounter Insect bite (nonvenomous) of right shoulder, subsequent encounter Insect bite (nonvenomous) of right shoulder, sequela

Abbreviation: *ICD-10-CM, International Classification of Diseases, 10th Revision, Clinical Modification.*

Figure 2-2 is an excerpt from the *ICD-10-CM* alphabetic index showing the starting point for finding the *ICD-10-CM* code for influenza—locating the main term, *influenza*, and sub-terms that lead to the most specific code category for the diagnosis of influenza with respiratory symptoms.

The main term *influenza* leads to sub-terms *with and respiratory manifestations* describing the cough and pharyngitis associated with the child's influenza. This directs you to reference code **J11.1** in the *ICD-10-CM* tabular list to verify the code is complete and any reporting instructions included in the tabular list.

After identifying code **J11.1** in the alphabetic index, turn to the code in the tabular list for more specific instructions. Coding instructions in the tabular list may appear at the chapter, block, category, subcategory, or code level, as illustrated in **Figure 2-3**.

- Code **J11.1** is in Chapter 10 and the block of codes **J09–J18**.
- An *ICD-10-CM* category is 3 characters (**J11** here) and may also be a code when no further characters are included in the tabular list.
  - > Category **J11** includes codes **J11.00–J11.89**.
  - > **J11.1** is a complete code (ie, no fifth characters are provided in subcategory **J11.1**).

Code level instructions at **J11.1** advise of other codes that should be reported when supported by the documented diagnosis (not supported by the example provided earlier).

> Use additional code for associated pleural effusion, if applicable (**J91.8**)
> Use additional code for associated sinusitis, if applicable (**J01.-**)

> Always see the instructions of the *ICD-10-CM* alphabetic index and tabular list when selecting a diagnosis code.

Figure 2-2. *ICD-10-CM* Alphabetic Index Example

> Words in parentheses are nonessential modifiers that do not affect code selection.

Influenza (bronchial) (epidemic) (respiratory [upper]) (unidentified influenza virus) J11.1

> This is a default code for the most common term or unspecified code for the condition. Use this when no more specific code is supported by the documentation.

- with

-- digestive manifestations **J11.2**

> The word *with* or *in* should be interpreted to mean "associated with" or "due to."

-- encephalopathy **J11.81**

-- enteritis **J11.2**

-- gastroenteritis **J11.2**

-- gastrointestinal manifestations **J11.2**

-- laryngitis **J11.1**

-- myocarditis **J11.82**

> *NEC* in the alphabetic index represents "other specified." Cough was specified in the diagnosis, but no code specifies influenza with cough. J11.1 is most specific to the diagnosis.

-- otitis media **J11.83**

-- pharyngitis **J11.1**

-- pneumonia **J11.00**

--- specified type **J11.08**

-- respiratory manifestations NEC **J11.1**

-- specified manifestation NEC **J11.89**

- A/H5N1 (*See also* Influenza, due to, identified novel influenza A virus) **J09.X2**

> Follow a *See also* instruction when the current entries do not provide the necessary code for a condition. Always follow a *See* instruction.

…

- due to

-- avian *See also* Influenza, due to, identified novel influenza A virus **J09.X2**

-- identified influenza virus NEC **J10.1**

--- with

-- identified novel influenza A virus **J09.X2**

> Had a specific novel influenza A virus been identified in the diagnosis, code J09.X2 would be referenced.

Abbreviations: *ICD-10-CM, International Classification of Diseases, 10th Revision, Clinical Modification*; NEC, not elsewhere classifiable.

Figure 2-3. Tabular List Respiratory System Chapter

Chapter 10: Diseases of the respiratory system (J00–J99)

Note: When a respiratory condition is described as occurring in more than one site and is not specifically indexed, it should be classified to the lower anatomic site (eg, tracheobronchitis to bronchitis in **J40**).

> Chapter notes such as this apply to the entire chapter.

Use additional code, where applicable, to identify:

> *Use additional code* notes are to be followed when applicable.

exposure to environmental tobacco smoke (**Z77.22**)

exposure to tobacco smoke in the perinatal period (**P96.81**)

history of tobacco dependence (**Z87.891**)

occupational exposure to environmental tobacco smoke (**Z57.31**)

tobacco dependence (**F17.-**)

tobacco use (**Z72.0**)

Excludes2: certain conditions originating in the perinatal period (**P04–P96**)

certain infectious and parasitic diseases (**A00–B99**)

...

congenital malformations, deformations and chromosomal abnormalities (**Q00–Q99**)

endocrine, nutritional and metabolic diseases (**E00–E88**)

injury, poisoning and certain other consequences of external causes (**S00–T88**)

neoplasms (**C00–D49**)

smoke inhalation (**T59.81-**)

symptoms, signs and abnormal clinical and laboratory findings, not elsewhere classified (**R00–R94**)

This chapter contains the following blocks:

J00–J06 Acute upper respiratory infections

J09–J18 Influenza and pneumonia

...

Influenza and pneumonia (J09–J18)

Excludes2: allergic or eosinophilic pneumonia (**J82**)

aspiration pneumonia NOS (**J69.0**)

meconium pneumonia (**P24.01**)

neonatal aspiration pneumonia (**P24.-**)

...

> Block note: An *Excludes2* note means "not included here." The codes in an *Excludes2* note may be additionally reported when applicable.

J11 Influenza due to unidentified influenza virus

> J11.1 is a complete code (no additional character applies).

...

J11.1 Influenza due to unidentified influenza virus with other respiratory manifestations

Influenza NOS

Influenzal laryngitis NOS

Influenzal pharyngitis NOS

Influenza with upper respiratory symptoms NOS

> Inclusion terms show some but not all conditions reported with this code. NOS = unspecified, documentation doesn't support a more specific code.

Use additional code for associated pleural effusion, if applicable (**J91.8**)

Use additional code for associated sinusitis, if applicable (**J01.-**)

J11.2 Influenza due to unidentified influenza virus with gastrointestinal manifestations

Influenza gastroenteritis NOS

> *Use additional code* is followed when useful to fully describe a condition.

Instructions at the beginning of a chapter in the tabular list apply to the entire chapter. For instance, Chapter 10 includes a *use additional code* note that instructs to report codes for exposure to or use of tobacco smoke when reporting any codes in the chapter.

Use additional code, where applicable, to identify:

exposure to environmental tobacco smoke (**Z77.22**)
exposure to tobacco smoke in the perinatal period (**P96.81**)

Based on this instruction, code **Z77.22** (or, in the case of exposure as a neonate, **P96.81**) would be reported in addition to influenza code **J11.1** because documentation indicates that child is currently exposed to tobacco smoke in the home.

Codes submitted for the child diagnosed with influenza with pharyngitis and cough with exposure to tobacco smoke in the home are as follows:

J11.1	Influenza due to unidentified influenza virus with other respiratory manifestations
Z77.22	Contact with and (suspected) exposure to environmental tobacco smoke (acute) (chronic)

Code Selection in an Electronic Health Record

Electronic health records (EHRs) often include *ICD-10-CM* codes chosen from drop-down lists. This is a quick method of code selection and usually effective for payment. However, *ICD-10-CM* code descriptors can be quite long and not fully display in the EHR. Depending how the inquiry is entered, the list may only give options for unspecified codes. This can be especially problematic when more details are required for proper coding. Also, commonly missing from EHR code selection tools are instructions included throughout the *ICD-10-CM* manual that are important to correct coding.

When you are aware of the instructions and conventions of *ICD-10-CM*, code lists and quick references can be improved to prompt more appropriate code selection. An ideal EHR selection tool will include full code descriptors and instructions from the *ICD-10-CM* manual.

Reporting *ICD-10-CM* Codes

Up to 12 *ICD-10-CM* codes may be reported per claim (listed in a claim field with labels A–L). However, only 4 diagnosis pointers (letters A–L from the diagnosis code field) can link the diagnoses to each procedure code reported.

See items 21 (fields labeled A–L for entry of *ICD-10-CM* codes) and 24E (diagnosis pointer) on the claim form example excerpt in **Figure 2-4**.

- For professional services, diagnosis codes are entered in the order listed in the documentation.
- The diagnosis that is chiefly responsible for the encounter is listed first.
- Linkage of multiple diagnoses to procedure codes is typically determined by the physician at the time of code selection or by coding staff following the encounter.

Figure 2-4. Example of Diagnosis Linking

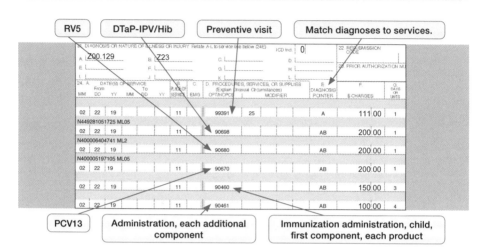

Abbreviations: DTaP, diphtheria, tetanus, acellular pertussis; Hib, *Haemophilus influenzae* type b; IPV, inactivated poliovirus; PCV13, pneumococcal conjugate; RV5, rotavirus.

It is important to correctly link diagnosis codes to services on the claim. If procedure code **99391** (preventive medicine evaluation and management [routine health examination] service) was linked only to diagnosis pointer B (code **Z23**, encounter for immunization), the charge for code **99391** may be denied for lack of a supporting diagnosis. Code **Z00.129** (encounter for routine child health examination without abnormal findings) is a more accurate diagnosis linkage to code **99391**.

ICD-10-CM instructs to code first any routine childhood examination (eg, **Z00.129**) when reporting code **Z23**.

Coding Keys

- It is important to begin an encounter by documenting the reason for the encounter, or *chief complaint.* The chief complaint leads to services and documentation of diagnoses. It might also be the final diagnosis at the end of the encounter.

- **Diagnosis codes explain a lot.** Diagnosis codes are used to report the reasons that services were provided. They should always be supported by documentation in the medical record. Be sure the *ICD-10-CM* code(s) selected are the most specific. Reserve "unspecified" codes only when appropriate.

- **Which code set is used for reporting diagnoses on health care claims?** *International Classification of Diseases, 10th Revision, Clinical Modification (ICD-10-CM).*

- **The *ICD-10-CM* manual contains 6 sections.**
  - > Official Guidelines for Coding and Reporting
  - > Alphabetic Index to Diseases and Injuries
  - > Table of Drugs and Chemicals
  - > Table of Neoplasms
  - > Index to External Causes of Injury
  - > Tabular List

- ***ICD-10-CM* code structure:** *ICD-10-CM* codes are 3 to 7 characters long. It is critical to always code to the highest level of specificity.
  - > The first character is a letter between A and Z.
  - > The second through seventh characters can be letters or numbers.
  - > Fourth through sixth characters indicate etiology, severity, site, manifestation(s) of an underlying etiology, or intent.

Resources

American Academy of Pediatrics

- *AAP Pediatric Coding Newsletter*™ (http://coding.aap.org)
- Coding Hotline (www.aap.org/en-us/Pages/cu/Coding-Hotline-Request.aspx)
- Coding Webinars (www.aap.org/en-us/professional-resources/practice-transformation/getting-paid/Coding-at-the-AAP/Pages/AAP-Coding-Webinars.aspx)

ICD-10-CM Code Files and Guidelines

- American Academy of Pediatrics *Pediatric ICD-10-CM: A Manual for Provider-Based Coding* (https://shop.aap.org)
- American Hospital Association *Coding Clinic* (https://www.codingclinicadvisor.com)
- National Center for Health Statistics *ICD-10-CM* (www.cdc.gov/nchs/icd/icd10cm.htm)

Coding Challenge

(Answers may be found in Appendix A.)

1. What does *ICD* stand for?

    a. *International Classification of Death*

    b. *International Classification of Diseases*

    c. *Independent Categorization of Disease*

    d. *Independent Classification of Diseases*

2. How many characters are placed to the left of the decimal point in an *International Classification of Diseases, 10th Revision, Clinical Modification (ICD-10-CM)* code?

    a. 7

    b. 3

    c. Up to 4

    d. 2

3. What letter is used to fill the fourth through sixth characters when necessary to support addition of a seventh character?

    a. X

    b. O

    c. None; a dash (-) is used.

    d. None; the seventh character is inserted in place of the fourth through sixth characters.

4. What claim item on the 1500 claim form is used to link diagnosis pointers to procedure codes?

    a. Item 21

    b. Item 24D

    c. Item 24E

    d. Item 24B

Chapter 3

Current Procedural Terminology®

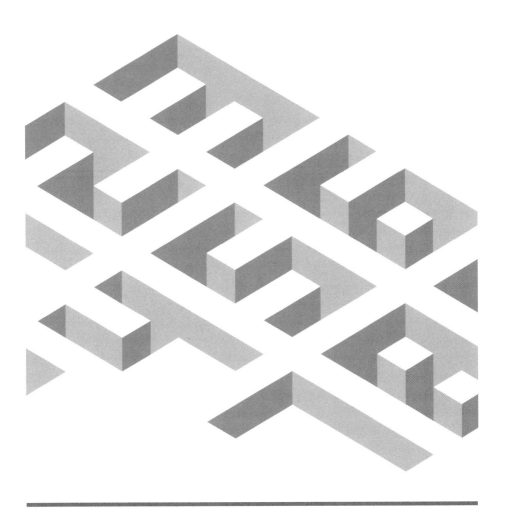

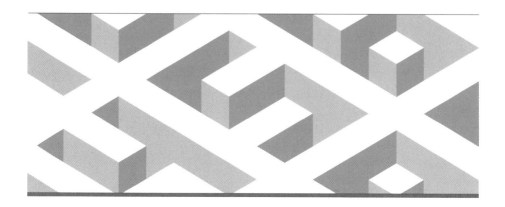

Coding Professional Services

Most professional services of pediatricians and other health care professionals (eg, advanced practice professionals) are reported using the American Medical Association (AMA) *Current Procedural Terminology (CPT®)* code set. **Table 3-1** provides an overview of the uses of the code set and effective dates.

Table 3-1. Overview of *Current Procedural Terminology (CPT®)* Codes	
Used to Report	**Effective Date**
• Most professional services	Annually, January 1
• Vaccine and immune globulin products • Tracking performance measurement	Exceptions: vaccine and Category III codes are implemented 6 months following the release date (eg, released July 1, implemented January 1).

CPT is also referred to as Level I of the Healthcare Common Procedure Coding System (HCPCS). However, most references to HCPCS are in relation to HCPCS Level II codes (discussed in Chapter 4), which are used primarily to report supplies and medications.

> ### *CPT* Code Development
>
> Anyone may submit an application to the *CPT* Editorial Panel to add, revise, or delete a *CPT* code. Collaboration with medical specialty organizations is strongly encouraged.

The AMA owns the copyright to *CPT* and oversees the processes of updating the code set annually. Anyone may propose a new or revised code, but collaboration with a medical specialty organization whose members will use the service represented by a code is recommended. The *CPT* Advisory Committee (physician members selected by their medical specialty organization and appointed by the AMA board) submits code change applications and/or reviews and comments on all code change applications for *CPT* Editorial Panel consideration prior to voting. The *CPT* Editorial Panel (physicians elected from participating specialties) vote to approve or deny code change applications.

The American Academy of Pediatrics (AAP) participates in the *CPT* update process with members selected by the AAP and appointed by the AMA board. These AAP members represent pediatrics on the *CPT* Advisory Committee.

Current Procedural Terminology (CPT) Categories, Sections, and Codes

CPT includes codes for

- **Category I** codes (includes the following sections)
  - > Evaluation and management (E/M) services (**99201–99499**) (eg, office visits, normal newborn care, critical care, emergency department services)
  - > Anesthesia (**01000–01999, 99100–99140**)

> *Current Procedural Terminology* begins with codes **99201–99499**? Yes, because evaluation and management services are the most frequently reported services.

> Surgery (**10004–69990**) (includes anatomical subsections)
> Radiology (**70010–79999**) (includes diagnostic, imaging guidance, oncology, radiation therapy)
> Pathology and laboratory (**80047–89398**, **0001U–0138U**)
> Medicine (**90281–99199**, **99500–99607**) (includes medical services not described in other sections, including immune globulins, serum, or recombinant products; vaccines; services provided by allied health professionals; and tests and therapeutic services other than radiology, pathology, or laboratory)

- **Category II** performance measurement codes (**0001F–9007F**)
- **Category III** temporary codes (**0042T–0593T**)

Codes are subject to revision or deletion periodically. The code ranges listed previously reflect code sections as of January 2020.

Categories

Category I Codes

- Represent the physician work entailed in evaluating and treating a patient as well as the practice expense and professional liability of the service.
- Consist of 5 digits (no alphabetical characters except in certain laboratory/pathology codes).
- Are updated and published annually. (If an urgent need to identify a service or vaccine product is identified, a code may be published for immediate or urgent release.)

Category I codes are assigned only for services that

- Are performed by most health care professionals, including pediatricians, in the United States.
- Are performed at a frequency consistent with clinical indications and current medical practice.
- The efficacy of the service is supported in medical literature.

If devices and drugs are necessary for the performance of the procedure or service, US Food and Drug Administration (FDA) approval of the devices and/or drugs is required for services described by Category I codes.

Services lacking any of these criteria are typically assigned a Category III code until a new application is presented showing that the service meets Category I criteria.

Category II Codes

- Are used to report performance measurement that supports nationally established performance measures and that has an evidence base that indicates it contributes to quality patient care.

- Are optional but will become more important to support quality initiatives and new payment initiatives that reward quality outcomes.

- An Alphabetical Clinical Topics Listing can be found on the AMA website (www.ama-assn.org/practice-management/cpt/criteria-cpt-category-ii-codes) and provides an overview of the measures to which each Category II code applies and reporting instructions.

Category III Codes

- Represent new services and/or emerging technologies for which the present medical literature and clinical experience do not yet meet the criteria required to be granted a Category I code. Payers may or may not pay for these services but commonly track utilization for future payment policy determination.

- Are released biannually with an implementation date 6 months following the release date. For instance, a code released on January 1, 2020, is implemented on July 1, 2020, and published in *CPT 2021*. The most recent Category III code listing is found at www.ama-assn.org/practice-management/category-iii-codes.

Symbols

CPT uses symbols to identify certain code properties (eg, new codes, revised codes). **Table 3-2** provides descriptions of each symbol.

Green font and triangles (▶◀) are used to identify text other than code descriptors that has been added or revised since the previous codebook was published.

Example

New instructions were added to the Introduction to *CPT 2020* under the Add-on Codes section.

▶ Add-on codes are always performed in addition to the primary service or procedure and must never be reported as a stand-alone code. When the add-on procedure can be reported bilaterally and is performed bilaterally, the appropriate add-on code is reported twice, unless the code descriptor, guidelines, or parenthetical instructions for that particular add-on code instructs otherwise. Do not report modifier **50**, Bilateral procedures, in conjunction with add-on codes. All add-on codes in the *CPT* code set are exempt from the multiple procedure concept. See the definitions of modifier **50** and **51** in Appendix A.◀

The symbols and font color draw attention to new instructions for reporting add-on codes for procedures performed bilaterally.

Table 3-2. Symbols and Descriptions in *CPT*	
Symbol	**Description**
•	A bullet at the beginning of a code means this is a new code for the current year (eg, •**95705** [new in *CPT 2020*]).
▲	A triangle means the code descriptor has been revised (eg, ▲**74022** [revised in *CPT 2020*]).
+	A plus sign means the code is an add-on code (eg, +**90461**, each additional vaccine or toxoid component administered [List separately in addition to code for primary procedure]).
⊘	A null sign means the code is a "modifier **51** exempt" code and, therefore, does not require modifier **51** (multiple procedures) even when reported with other procedures (eg, ⊘**94610**, intrapulmonary surfactant administration by a physician or other qualified health care professional through endotracheal tube).
#	The pound symbol is used to identify re-sequenced codes that are out of numerical sequence. This allows related codes to be placed in an appropriate section of codes when consecutive numbers are not available.
⚡	The lightning bolt identifies codes for vaccines that are pending US Food and Drug Administration approval (eg, ⚡**90668**, influenza virus vaccine [IIV], pandemic formulation, split virus, for intramuscular use).
★	A star means the service represented by the code is included in Appendix P of the *CPT* manual as a code to which modifier **95** (synchronous telemedicine service) may be appended to indicate the service was rendered via real-time telemedicine services.
Mutiple	Some codes may have more than one symbol (eg, #⚡•**90619**—re-sequenced, not yet FDA approved, and a new code).

Abbreviations: *CPT*, *Current Procedural Terminology*; FDA, US Food and Drug Administration.

CPT Code Structure and Conventions

CPT is structured to save space in the listing of codes by use of indentations to identify variations of services that have a common base descriptor.

Example

90460	**Immunization administration through 18 years of age via any route of administration, with counseling by physician or other qualified health care professional;** first or only component of each vaccine or toxoid administered
+**90461**	each additional vaccine or toxoid component administered (List separately in addition to code for primary procedure) (Use **90460** for each vaccine administered. For vaccines with multiple components [combination vaccines], report **90460** in conjunction with **90461** for each additional component in a given vaccine.)

The portion of the code descriptor for **90460** before the semicolon also applies to code **90461**. Increased indentation of codes that share a portion of the first code's descriptor helps to identify which codes share a common base procedure.

Code **90461** is an add-on code symbolized by a plus (+) sign in *CPT*. Add-on codes are used when you provide the primary procedure (eg, counseling and administration of the first component of a vaccine) and the service described by the add-on code (eg, counseling and administration of each additional vaccine component). Parenthetical instructions following add-on codes provide a listing of primary codes with which the add-on code is reported.

As code sections expand, new codes may be added between consecutive code numbers or out of numerical sequence. Codes placed out of numerical sequence are identified by a pound or hashtag symbol (#) preceding the code.

Example

Subsequent observation care codes 99224–99226 are placed between codes 99220 (initial observation care, level three) and 99221 (initial hospital care, level one). Codes with notes follow code **99223** (initial hospital care, level three), indicating where the re-sequenced codes with descriptors are located.

> **Add-on Codes**
>
> Add-on codes, identified by a plus (+) sign, are used to report procedures commonly carried out in addition to a primary procedure. Parenthetical instructions following add-on codes provide a listing of primary codes with which the add-on code is reported.

99224 Code is out of numerical sequence. See **99219–99222**

99225 Code is out of numerical sequence. See **99219–99222**

99226 Code is out of numerical sequence. See **99219–99222**

Code Descriptors

Code descriptors specify the type and, when applicable, extent of service.

- Descriptors may include specific work elements (eg, collection of blood by venipuncture versus capillary stick) or characteristics of the patient (eg, age).

- Some codes denote specific time ranges that must be met to report the code; other codes simply note a typical time health care professionals spend in completing the service.

Most E/M codes also include a patient admission status or site of service (eg, inpatient hospital, observation, emergency department).

Example

Some codes are reported per day of service, meaning they can only be reported once on any date of service. Management of a normal newborn is reported daily (initial day is also based on site of service and whether or not the patient is discharged on the same date).

99460	Initial hospital or birthing center care, per day, for evaluation and management of normal newborn infant
99461	Initial care, per day, for evaluation and management of normal newborn infant seen in *other than* hospital or birthing center
99462	Subsequent hospital care, per day, for evaluation and management of normal newborn
99463	Initial hospital or birthing center care, per day, for evaluation and management of normal newborn infant admitted and discharged on the same date
	(For newborn hospital discharge services provided on a date subsequent to the admission date, see **99238**, **99239**)

Some codes include specific time requirements.

99291	Critical care, evaluation and management of the critically ill or critically injured patient; first 30-74 minutes

Some codes may be reported based on specific work elements or on time (when certain requirements are met).

99221	Initial hospital care, per day, for the evaluation and management of a patient, which requires these 3 key components:

- A detailed or comprehensive history;
- A detailed or comprehensive examination; and
- Medical decision making that is straightforward or of low complexity.

> **Evaluation and Management Key Components**
>
> The key components (ie, history, examination, and medical decision-making) are defined in guidelines for evaluation and management services.

Counseling and/or coordination of care with other physicians, other qualified health care professionals, or agencies are provided consistent with the nature of the problem(s) and the patient's and/or family's needs.

Usually, the problem(s) requiring admission are of low severity. Typically, *30 minutes* are spent at the bedside and on the patient's hospital floor or unit.

Two Code-Selection Options for Certain Evaluation and Management Services

Evaluation and management services that are assigned key components and a typical time may be reported based on time (in lieu of key components) when more than 50% of the reporting pediatrician's time was spent providing care to the individual patient either face-to-face with the patient/caregiver or, in a facility setting, on the unit or floor.

Some codes are reported based on multiple factors (eg, approach, with or without anesthesia, patient age).

54150	Circumcision, using clamp or other device with regional dorsal penile or ring block
54160	Circumcision, surgical excision other than clamp, device, or dorsal slit; neonate (28 days of age or less)
54161	older than 28 days of age
24300	Manipulation, elbow, under anesthesia

The code descriptors, in conjunction with guidelines and instructions, provide details necessary for selecting the code that describes a specific service.

Modifiers

Modifiers are also part of the *CPT* code set. Modifiers help identify special circumstances that apply when a service was provided. *CPT* modifiers are 2 digits (eg, **50**, bilateral procedure). Modifiers often affect whether a health plan pays or does not pay for a service. Some modifiers commonly used in pediatric coding are included in **Table 3-3**.

Not all modifiers affect payment. Some modifiers are generally considered informational. Payers often publish information on which modifiers affect payment and which are informational only (eg, **47**, anesthesia by surgeon).

Modifiers are also part of the HCPCS Level II code set. *CPT* and HCPCS modifiers are not limited to use with codes in the same HCPCS level. For instance, HCPCS modifier **TC** (technical component) is used to indicate that only the technical component of a service was provided by the reporting individual/facility; another individual may report the same code with modifier **26** (professional component).

Table 3-3. Select *CPT* Modifiers		
Modifier	**Brief Description of Modifier**	**Example**
24	Unrelated E/M service by the same physician or other qualified health care professional during a postoperative period	**99213 24** An office visit (for a reason unrelated to a recent procedure) meeting the requirements for **99213** is provided within the global period of a procedure (eg, within 90 days of a major procedure).
25	Significant, separately identifiable E/M service by the same physician or other qualified health care professional on the same day of the procedure or other service	**99214 25** A patient presents for a preventive E/M service and a significant E/M service to address a problem is provided and distinctly documented.
26	Professional component	**73100 26** A physician interprets 2 views of the wrist, but another party is billing for the technical work of producing the images.
33	Preventive services	**80061 33** A lipid panel is performed to screen for lipid disorders in a patient with no symptoms.
50	Bilateral procedure	**73100 50** A patient has bilateral wrist injuries. Radiographs of each wrist are obtained with interpretation and report by the same party.
59	Distinct procedural service	**10120, 10120 59** Two different body areas are incised with removal of foreign bodies.
63	Procedures performed on infants less than 4 kg	**93530 26 63** Combined right heart catheterization and retrograde left heart catheterization, for congenital cardiac anomalies performed on an infant with present body weight of less than 4 kg (professional component only)

Abbreviations: *CPT, Current Procedural Terminology;* E/M, evaluation and management.

The *CPT* Codebook

CPT is available in print and electronic formats (eg, applications, freestanding software, data files embedded in other software). Regardless of the format by which codes are selected, it is important to reference more than a list of the procedure codes.

Beyond codes, *CPT* includes important instructions for use of the codebook, section guidelines, and instructions at code categories and following individual codes. If you are not aware of the guidelines and instructions of *CPT*, you may erroneously report a code that appears correct based on its descriptor alone.

Example

You see a 5-day-old for a well-child (health supervision) check. Another pediatrician in your group practice provided hospital care to the newborn during the birth admission. You might select code **99381**.

99381	Initial comprehensive preventive medicine evaluation and management of an individual including an age and gender appropriate history, examination, counseling/anticipatory guidance/risk factor reduction interventions, and the ordering of laboratory/diagnostic procedures, new patient; infant (age younger than 1 year)

This code is *incorrect* because **99381** is a code for a new patient encounter. The *CPT* guidelines for E/M services define a new patient as one who has not received a face-to-face professional service *from you or another physician of the same exact specialty and same group practice* (billing entity defined by tax identification number) *in the past 3 years*. Your patient has received face-to-face professional services while hospitalized from a physician of the same exact specialty and group practice and, therefore, is an established patient for your services. The correct code is **99391**.

99391	Periodic comprehensive preventive medicine reevaluation and management of an individual including an age and gender appropriate history, examination, counseling/anticipatory guidance/risk factor reduction interventions, and the ordering of laboratory/diagnostic procedures, established patient; infant (age younger than 1 year)

General Instructions

The first and perhaps most important instruction for use of the *CPT* codebook is as follows:

> An *unlisted* procedure code is a nonspecific code indicating only the general nature of a service.
>
> **Example: 99499**, unlisted evaluation and management service

Select the name of the procedure or service that accurately identifies the service performed. Do not select a *CPT* code that merely approximates the service provided. If no specific code exists, report with an unlisted procedure or service code. (In some cases, a modifier may be used to indicate a reduced, discontinued, or increased procedural service in lieu of an unlisted procedure code.)

Other important general instructions include

- When advanced practice nurses and physician assistants are working with physicians, they are considered to be working in the exact same specialty and exact same subspecialties as the physician.

- Some *CPT* descriptors specifically require interpretation and reporting of test results to report that code. These codes are not reported for review of another individual's report of test results.

- *CPT* distinguishes a physician or other qualified health care professional (QHP) from clinical staff.

> A physician or QHP is an individual who is qualified by education, training, licensure, or regulation (when applicable), and facility privileging (when applicable), who performs a professional service within his or her scope of practice and independently reports that professional service.

> A clinical staff member is a person who works under the supervision of a physician or other QHP and who is allowed by law, regulation, and facility policy to perform or assist in the performance of a specified professional service but who does not individually report that professional service.

Types of *CPT* Instructions

In addition to guidelines provided for each section of *CPT*, other types of instructions include the following:

- Prefatory instructions precede many code categories.
- Coding Tips are provided in certain sections, often repeating related guidelines found elsewhere.
- Instructions in parentheses follow many codes (examples follow).

Examples

94060	Bronchodilation responsiveness, spirometry as in **94010**, pre- and post-bronchodilator administration
	(Do not report **94060** in conjunction with **94150**, **94200**, **94375**, **94640**, **94728**)
	(Report bronchodilator supply separately with **99070** or appropriate supply code)
	(For exercise test for bronchospasm with pre- and post-spirometry, use **94617**)

Each parenthetical instruction applies to the code that immediately precedes the instructions.

In addition to instructions in the *CPT* codebook, the AMA publishes *CPT Assistant*, a monthly subscription-based publication that offers articles that provide additional guidance for correct coding. Although not authoritative to health plans, *CPT Assistant* is often used to support health plan payment policies.

Appendixes in *CPT* provide clinical examples of E/M services; quick references to modifiers; a summary of new, revised, and deleted codes; add-on and modifier-exempt codes; and other procedure code references. Based on changes to the coding manual, the appendixes may vary from year to year. **Table 3-4** lists the appendixes included in *CPT 2020*.

Table 3-4. *CPT* Appendixes[a]	
Symbols	**Description**
Appendix A	A list of all modifiers applicable to current-year codes
Appendix B	A listing of all new codes, revised codes with markup showing revisions to the code descriptors (ie, new text <u>underlined</u>, deleted text ~~struck through~~), and newly deleted codes
Appendix C	Clinical examples developed by physicians of various specialties are provided for office or other outpatient services, hospital inpatient services, consultations, critical care, prolonged services, and care plan oversight E/M codes. Examples provide only typical patients with problems that may commonly require each type of service. Codes are selected based on the actual work performed and documented for each encounter.
Appendix D	A listing of all add-on codes
Appendix E	A listing of all procedure codes that are exempt from modifier **51** when the same physician is reporting another procedure on the same date. Procedures represented by these codes are typically performed with other procedures but may be stand-alone procedures as well.
Appendix F	Codes listed here are not reported with modifier **63** (procedure performed on neonates and infants up to a present body weight of 4 kg). Services represented by these codes are valued to reflect the intensity required when performed on patients weighing 4 kg or less.
Appendix J	This is a summary of each sensory, motor, and mixed nerve listed with its appropriate nerve conduction study code to enhance accurate reporting of codes **95907–95913**.
Appendix K	Each vaccine code that, at time of publication, was not yet FDA-approved (✔ is appended to these codes in the vaccine code section).
Appendix L	To aid with selection of codes for vascular catheterization, vascular families are listed starting with either the aorta, vena cava, pulmonary artery, or portal vein.
Appendix M	This is a list of codes that were deleted and renumbered from 2007 to 2009. *CPT* no longer deletes and renumbers codes, so this list does not change from year to year.
Appendix N	Tables of codes that are re-sequenced (appear out of sequence) are listed along with the corresponding code range where the re-sequenced codes appear. These are codes preceded by the # symbol.
Appendix O	A listing of 3 types of codes for multianalyte assays with algorithmic analyses; this list includes a proprietary name and clinical laboratory or manufacturer in the first column, an alphanumeric code in the second column, and a code descriptor in the third column.
Appendix P	This is a list of codes that may be reported with modifier **95** (synchronous telemedicine service rendered via a real-time interactive audio and video telecommunications system) when provided via telemedicine.

Abbreviations: *CPT, Current Procedural Terminology;* E/M, evaluation and management; FDA, US Food and Drug Administration.

[a] Appendixes are subject to change. Listing is current with *CPT 2020.*

Selecting Codes

There are more than 10,000 codes to choose from in *CPT*. An alphabetical index is used to find codes and/or code ranges to help guide the user to the correct section(s) of codes.

- Codes should not be selected from the index without verification in the main text of the manual (numerical listing).
- Terms in the index include services, organs and anatomical sites, conditions, synonyms, eponyms, and abbreviations (eg, EEG [electroencephalogram]).

Table 3-5 provides examples from the *CPT* index.

Table 3-5. Selecting Codes: Examples From *CPT* Index
Myringotomy 69420, 69421
New Patient Domiciliary or Rest Home Visit **99324–99328** Emergency Department Services **99281–99288** Home Services **99341–99345** Hospital Inpatient Services **99221–99239** Hospital Observation Services **99217–99220** Initial Office Visit **99201–99205** Inpatient Consultations **99251–99255** Office and/or Other Outpatient Consultations **99241–99245**

Frenum
Lip
   Excision **40819**
   Incision **40806**
Tongue
   Excision **41115**
   Incision **41010**
Revision **41520**

Norwood Procedure 33611, 33612, 33619 See Repair, Heart, Ventricle; Revision
MAGPI Operation 54322

Cerumen
Removal
   with Instrumentation **69210**
   with Irrigation/Lavage **69209**

[a] Abbreviation: MAGPI, meatal advancement and glanuloplasty.

Once you have selected a code or code range from the alphabetical index, it is always necessary to consult the numerical listing for the code(s) to select the appropriate code(s) for reporting a service using the guidelines and instructions for the code section.

Example

You have repaired a patent ductus arteriosus (PDA) via percutaneous transcatheter closure. You look in the alphabetical index and find the following reference:

Arteriosus, Ductus
Closure

> Transcatheter Percutaneous **93582**

(You could also look under "Ductus, arteriosus, closure"; "Patent Ductus Arteriosus (PDA), repair"; or "Repair, patent ductus arteriosus.")

You turn to code 93582 in the numerical listing and find the code is followed by a number of parenthetical instructions.

93582	Percutaneous transcatheter closure of patent ductus arteriosus
	(**93582** includes congenital right and left heart catheterization, catheter placement in the aorta, and aortic arch angiography, when performed)
	(Do not report **93582** in conjunction with **36013, 36014, 36200, 75600, 75605, 93451–93461, 93530, 93531, 93532, 93533, 93567**)
	(For other cardiac angiographic procedures performed at the time of transcatheter PDA closure, see **93563, 93564, 93565, 93566, 93568** as appropriate)
	(For left heart catheterization by transseptal puncture through intact septum or by transapical puncture performed at the time of transcatheter PDA closure, use **93462**)
	(For repair of patent ductus arteriosus by ligation, see **33820, 33822, 33824**)
	(For intracardiac echocardiographic services performed at the time of transcatheter PDA closure, use **93662**. Other echocardiographic services provided by a separate individual are reported using the appropriate echocardiography service codes, **93315, 93316, 93317**)

Each of the parenthetical instructions is important to accurately reporting all your services on the date of this procedure. For example, you would not separately report cardiac catheterization for congenital cardiac anomalies (**93530–93533**) performed at the time of closure of the PDA. However, code **+93568** (injection procedure during cardiac catheterization including imaging supervision, interpretation, and report; for pulmonary angiography) may be reported in addition to code **93582**, when performed.

Once you have gained familiarity with *CPT*, many codes may be selected by going to the appropriate section of the numerical list. However, it is best to always verify the code selection options in the alphabetical index so that you are fully aware of all codes that may apply.

General Tips and Principles for Reporting *CPT* Codes

Now that you have learned about *CPT* codes and how to find them in the codebook, it may be helpful to learn a few basic tips and principles for reporting *CPT* codes.

Use up-to-date references. *CPT* changes annually, including changes to codes and reporting instructions. Always invest in and use a current codebook or reference.

Codes are not limited by placement in *CPT*. Any individual whose license and credentialing allow performance of a service may report the code for that service. For instance, a primary care pediatrician might report a procedure found in a surgical subsection of codes.

Select codes based on documentation. Codes must always be supported by documentation. Documentation must include information that supports the code, including, but not limited to

- The date of service
- Reason(s) service was indicated
- Findings and assessment or impression
- Measurements (eg, centimeter length of wound repair, width of wound)
- Time (when time based)
- Clinical detail sufficient to differentiate one service from another
- The authentication of the individual documenting the service, including name and credentials

> **_CPT_ codes must be supported by *ICD-10-CM* codes reflecting the reason services were indicated.**

Use of Time in Code Selection

- In general, time references in *CPT* apply to a physician or other QHP's face-to-face time with the patient in a non-facility setting or the time on the patient's unit or floor in a facility setting.
- Codes that apply to non–face-to-face time or clinical staff time are designated as such in the code descriptors and instructions.
- For reporting purposes, time of service is met for time-based codes when the midpoint is passed ("midpoint rule") unless otherwise stated (eg, a service stated as 15 minutes is reported when at least 8 minutes of service is documented).
  - > Specific time ranges or minimum times may be stated in a code descriptor and are not overridden by the midpoint rule.
  - > Prefatory or parenthetical instructions may also override the midpoint rule.

Bilateral Procedures

Some services may be provided on body parts unilaterally or bilaterally. It is important to follow instruction when reporting these procedures.

Examples

Code 61000 is reported with 1 unit of service whether performed unilaterally or bilaterally. This is indicated by inclusion of "unilateral or bilateral" in the code descriptor.

61000	Subdural tap through fontanelle, or suture, infant, unilateral or bilateral; initial

Code 54550 represents a unilateral procedure. Parenthetical instruction that follows the code instructs to append modifier 50 (bilateral service) when the procedure is performed bilaterally.

54550	Exploration for undescended testis (inguinal or scrotal area)
	(For bilateral procedure, report 54550 with modifier 50)

Codes 55040 and 55041 designate whether an excision of hydrocele was unilateral or bilateral. It would be inaccurate to report 55040 with modifier 50.

55040	Excision of hydrocele; unilateral
55041	bilateral

When appending modifier **50** to indicate a bilateral procedure, 1 unit of service is reported unless a health plan policy requires otherwise. Because of overlap of some of the preservice and post-service work of bilateral procedures, health plans typically allow 150% of the unilateral fee schedule amount for procedures performed bilaterally.

With or Without Anesthesia

Some code descriptors include phrases such as "with anesthesia" or "without anesthesia." This is not an indication that anesthesia, other than local anesthesia, is not separately billed. The terms *with anesthesia* and *without anesthesia* are used to indicate the complexity of the procedure.

Example

27093	Injection procedure for hip arthrography; without anesthesia
27095	with anesthesia

Local anesthesia is included in surgical procedures and not separately reported. Do not report a code that includes "with anesthesia" in the descriptor when only local anesthesia was required.

Coding Keys

- *Current Procedural Terminology (CPT)* codes are used for
  - > Most professional services
  - > Vaccines and immune globulin products
  - > Tracking performance measurement
- There are 3 categories of *CPT* codes. Here is what is included in each category.
  - > **Category I:** evaluation and management (E/M), anesthesia, surgery, radiology, pathology and laboratory, and medicine codes
  - > **Category II:** performance measurement codes
  - > **Category III:** temporary codes
- Code descriptors specify type and, when applicable, extent of service. They can include specific work elements or characteristics of the patient. Some denote specific time ranges that must be met to report the code, while others note the typical time that health care professionals spend completing the service. Most E/M codes also include a patient admission status or site of service.
- *CPT* modifiers play an important role. Modifiers are 2 digits long and help identify special circumstances that apply when a service is provided (eg, bilateral procedure or preventive services).
- When to use an unlisted procedure or service code: An unlisted procedure or service code is used when specific codes that accurately identify the service performed do not exist. In some cases, a modifier might be used to indicate a reduced, discontinued, or increased procedural service in lieu of an unlisted procedure code.

Resources

American Academy of Pediatrics

- *AAP Pediatric Coding Newsletter*™ (http://coding.aap.org)
- Coding Webinars (www.aap.org/en-us/professional-resources/practice-transformation/getting-paid/Coding-at-the-AAP/Pages/AAP-Coding-Webinars.aspx)

Bilateral Procedure Identification

- Medicare Physician Fee Schedule Relative Value Files (www.cms.gov/Medicare/Medicare-Fee-for-Service-Payment/PhysicianFeeSched/PFS-Relative-Value-Files.html; see Column Z [BILAT SURG] in file applicable to date of service)

Current Procedural Terminology

- American Academy of Pediatrics *Coding for Pediatrics* (www.aap.org/cfp)
- American Medical Association *CPT* general information (www.ama-assn.org/practice-management/cpt-current-procedural-terminology)
- Category II code changes (www.ama-assn.org/practice-management/category-ii-codes)
- Category III code list (www.ama-assn.org/practice-management/category-iii-codes)

National Correct Coding Initiative (NCCI) Edits

- American Academy of Pediatrics NCCI file links (www.aap.org/coding; see the "Coding Resources, National Correct Coding Initiative (NCCI) Edits" tab)
- Medicaid NCCI website (www.medicaid.gov/medicaid/program-integrity/national-correct-coding-initiative-medicaid/index.html)
- Medicare NCCI website (www.cms.gov/NationalCorrectCodInitEd/NCCIEP/list.asp)

National Drug Codes

- US Food and Drug Administration National Drug Code Directory (www.fda.gov/drugs/informationondrugs/ucm142438.htm)

Coding Challenge

(Answers may be found in Appendix A.)

1. In which *Current Procedural Terminology* (*CPT*) appendix will you find a listing of modifiers?

    a. Appendix A

    b. Appendix B

    c. Appendix M

    d. Appendix X

2. Which of the following is not a criterion for Category I creation in *CPT*?

    a. Paid by many health plans

    b. Performed by most health care professionals, including pediatricians, in the United States

    c. Performed at a frequency consistent with clinical indications and current medical practice

    d. The efficacy of the service is supported in medical literature.

3. A code preceded by a plus sign (+) is

    a. A new code

    b. An add-on code

    c. A code for new or emerging technology

    d. A service that may be provided via telemedicine

4. When selecting a *CPT* code, which of the following is true?

    a. Codes should be selected from the alphabetical index alone.

    b. A code that approximates the service provided is sufficient.

    c. Never select an unlisted procedure code.

    d. Use the guidelines and instructions in the numerical listing to guide code selection.

Chapter 4

Healthcare Common Procedure Coding System and National Drug Codes

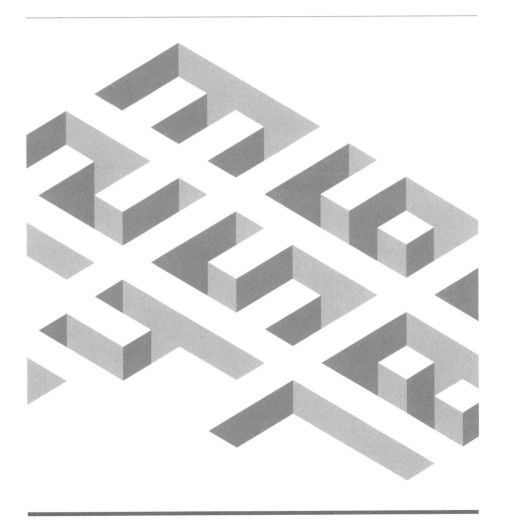

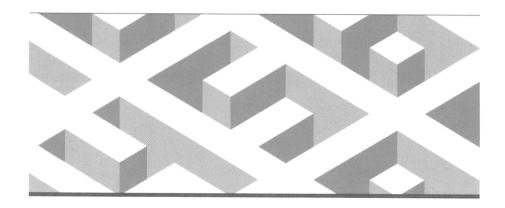

Healthcare Common Procedure Coding System (HCPCS)

Level II Healthcare Common Procedure Coding System (HCPCS) codes are used to describe supplies, products, and services not described by *Current Procedural Terminology* (*CPT®*) (HCPCS Level I) codes. In this chapter, HCPCS refers to HCPCS Level II codes. **Table 4-1** provides an overview of HCPCS code uses and effective dates.

Pediatricians often report these codes for injectable medications administered in an office setting and supplies such as slings, splints, or orthotics (eg, walking boot) provided in an office setting. Certain services not described by *CPT* are also included in HCPCS.

Table 4-1. Healthcare Common Procedure Coding System (HCPCS) Overview	
Used to Report	**Effective Date**
• Supplies • Medications • Services (when a *CPT* code does not describe the service as covered by health plan benefits)	Annually, January 1 Exceptions: quarterly updates for temporary codes

Abbreviation: *CPT, Current Procedural Terminology.*

HCPCS Codes

HCPCS codes are alphanumeric with a letter followed by 4 numbers.

Examples of HCPCS Codes

Q4011	Cast supplies, short arm cast, pediatric [0-10 years], plaster
J0696	Injection, ceftriaxone sodium, per 250 mg
S0630	Removal of sutures by a physician other than the physician who originally closed the wound

> **Supply Codes for Casts**
>
> *Current Procedural Terminology* (*CPT*) codes for fracture care include the first cast/splint or strap application. Healthcare Common Procedure Coding System codes are not reported when reporting *CPT* fracture care codes.

Some HCPCS codes, like **S0630**, describe physician services. To determine whether to report a HCPCS or *CPT* code, consider the following:

- Choose a HCPCS code when no *CPT* code adequately describes the service or as required by a specific health plan.
- When both a *CPT* and a HCPCS Level II code have the same descriptor, use the *CPT* code unless a health plan requires the HCPCS code.

Some HCPCS codes describe supply items that are already included in the practice expense value assigned to the *CPT* code describing a particular service (eg, tubing, surgical trays).

When a health plan pays separately for supplies used to provide a service, verify whether the plan requires reporting of HCPCS codes or *CPT* code **99070**.

99070	Supplies and materials (except spectacles), provided by the physician or other qualified health care professional over and above those usually included with the office visit or other services rendered (list drugs, trays, supplies, or materials provided)

The Centers for Medicare & Medicaid Services (CMS) maintains the HCPCS code set. The CMS has the flexibility to add, change, or discontinue temporary codes on a quarterly basis. Newly established temporary codes are usually implemented within 90 days of publication. Otherwise, HCPCS codes are updated annually on January 1.

> Health plans that pay based on relative value units will not pay separately for supplies commonly used to provide a service.

Using a HCPCS Manual

HCPCS codes are grouped in sections based on the type of product or service described (**Table 4-2**). A HCPCS manual also includes an

- Alphabetical index
- Table of drugs
- List of modifiers

Features of Some HCPCS Manuals

Nearly all HCPCS manuals place references to the Medicare policy manual (Pub. 100 references) beneath codes that are addressed in the manuals. Many also include references to the subscription-based American Hospital Association (AHA) *Coding Clinic for HCPCS* articles under each code that has been addressed in a particular article. Users who have access to *Coding Clinic for HCPCS* can use these references to find guidance on use of the related code.

Many HCPCS manuals include features to help physicians and coders identify codes that have specific coverage or payment indications. Assignment of these features is often based on the policies of the Medicare Outpatient Prospective Payment System (OPPS), which is not applicable to professional services. However, other health plans may adopt policies of the OPPS.

Symbols or colored blocks around codes are often used to indicate

- Age or sex limitations may apply (based on edits developed for Medicare).
- Ambulatory Surgery Center (ASC) payment and status indicators.
- Durable medical equipment, orthotics, prosthetics, and supply payment indicators.
- Indicators of the number of billing units reportable under payment policy.
- Indication of codes used for participation in Medicare quality measurement initiatives.

Table 4-2. HCPCS Code Manual Sections	
Section	**Codes[a]**
Ambulance and other transport services and supplies	A0021–A0999
Medical and surgical supplies	A4206–A8004
Administrative, miscellaneous, and investigational	A9150–A9999
Enteral and parenteral therapy	B4034–B9999
CMS hospital outpatient prospective payment system	C1713–C9899
DME	E0100–E8002
Temporary procedures/professional services	G0008–G9987
Behavioral health and/or substance abuse treatments services (used by state Medicaid plans to meet requirements of state law)	H0001–H2037
Drugs other than oral method; chemotherapy	J0120–J8999; J9000–J9999
Temporary codes assigned to DME regional carriers	K0001–K0900
Orthotics procedures and services; prosthetic procedures	L0112–L4631; L5000–L9900
Other medical services; screening procedures	M0075–M0301; M1000–M1071
Pathology and laboratory services	P2028–P9615
Temporary codes assigned by CMS (many used long-term)	Q0035–Q9995
Diagnostic radiology services	R0070–R0076
Temporary national codes established by private payers	S0012–S9999
Temporary national codes established by Medicaid agencies	T1000–T5999
Vision services; hearing services	V5008–V2799; V5008–V5364

Abbreviations: CMS, Centers for Medicare & Medicaid Services; DME, durable medical equipment; HCPCS, Healthcare Common Procedure Coding System.

[a] Code ranges were current as of HCPCS 2020 and are subject to change. Please see a current HCPCS manual for current codes.

Modifiers

HCPCS contains an extensive list of modifiers that may be used in conjunction with either HCPCS or *CPT* codes. HCPCS modifiers are 2 characters that may contain numbers and letters and are used to report specific information not conveyed in code descriptors or by *CPT* modifiers, such as

E1	Upper left eyelid
QW	Performance of tests waived by Clinical Laboratory Improvement Amendments (CLIA)
RT	Right side
TC	Technical component only
XE	Procedural services performed at separate encounters on the same date

Examples

You order, and your staff performs, a laboratory test that has waived status under CLIA.

Modifier **QW** is appended to the *CPT* code for the test.

You treat a fracture of the left second finger.

The code for treating the fracture is reported with modifier **F1** (left hand, second digit). Modifiers identifying body sites or laterality can be important should a patient have multiple injuries treated and/or require multiple services to different body sites.

> What is Clinical Laboratory Improvement Amendments (CLIA)? CLIA is a federal program requiring all laboratories to be certified and show proficiency in testing.

You perform the interpretation of a test that was performed in a hospital.

Your professional service is reported with the appropriate *CPT* code appended with *CPT* modifier **26** (professional component). The hospital reports the same *CPT* code with modifier **TC** (technical component) to receive payment for the expense of providing the test (eg, equipment, supplies, technician).

You perform a procedure early in the day. Later on the same date, you perform another procedure on the same patient. Health plan policy indicates that only the first procedure is paid when both procedures are performed at the same encounter.

You append modifier **XE** to the code for the second procedure on the same date to indicate the services were provided at separate encounters.

Finding HCPCS Codes

Things to know when using a HCPCS manual include

- For supplies or services other than drugs, the alphabetical index is typically the easiest starting point for locating a code. Searchable electronic applications are often more user-friendly for locating HCPCS codes.
- Drugs are more easily found by referencing the Table of Drugs in which one can search by brand or generic drug name, dose per unit billed, and route of administration (eg, injection, inhalation).

- The code descriptions may include any one of the following terms for nonspecific codes:

  > Unlisted

  > Not otherwise classified (NOC)

  > Unspecified

  > Unclassified

  > Other and miscellaneous

Selecting Codes for Supplies and Services

The alphabetical index provides a quick reference to most codes. However, if a term is not indexed, it may be necessary to think of another term for the same supply or service. For some supplies, the HCPCS index may guide you only to the section of codes from which you can choose a specific code.

Examples

You provide a patient with a finger splint in your office and report an office visit for evaluation and management of the related injury.

Q4049   Finger splint, static

You may or may not find a HCPCS index entry for a finger splint under *finger* or *splint* in your HCPCS manual. If not, cross-reference to *cast supplies*, where you are directed to **Q4049**.

Alphabetical Index Excerpt: Cast

- Hand restoration **L6900–L6915**
- Materials, special **A4590**
- Supplies
  -- Body
  -- Fiberglass **A4590**
  -- Finger splint, static **Q4049**

You provide a patient with a pneumatic walking boot to protect his ankle following an injury.

Alphabetical Index Excerpt: Pneumatic

- Appliance **E0655–E0673, L4350–L4370**

The term *boot* may lead only to "pelvic, **E0944**" and "surgical, ambulatory, **L3260**." However, the term *pneumatic* leads to "appliance, **L4350–L4370**." Looking at codes **L4350–L4370**, you find 2 codes for walking boots.

L4360	Walking boot, pneumatic and/or vacuum, with or without joints, with or without interface material, prefabricated item that has been trimmed, bent, molded, assembled, or otherwise customized to fit a specific patient by an individual with expertise
L4361	Walking boot, pneumatic and/or vacuum, with or without joints, with or without interface material, prefabricated, off-the-shelf

Code **L4361** describes the off-the-shelf pneumatic walking boot supplied.

A quick-pick list, either in your electronic health record or as a separate quick reference tool, can facilitate easier code assignment for common supplies and services reported with HCPCS codes. However, such lists must be routinely updated.

> ### HCPCS Coding Quick Reference
>
> A quick-pick list, either in your electronic health record or as a separate quick reference tool, can facilitate easier code assignment for common supplies and services reported with Healthcare Common Procedure Coding System codes. However, such lists must be routinely updated.

Selecting Codes for Medications

Medications are typically not included in charges for administration (eg, bill a *CPT* code for administration by injection and a HCPCS code for the medication supplied by the practice). The HCPCS Table of Drugs is a quick way to locate the code for a medication. The Table of Drugs describes route of administration using the following abbreviations:

IA: Intra-arterial administration

IM: Intramuscular administration

INH: Administration by inhaled solution

IT: Intrathecal

IV: Intravenous administration (includes all methods, such as gravity infusion, injections, and timed pushes)

ORAL: Administered orally

OTH: Other routes of administration (indicates other administration methods, such as suppositories or catheter injections)

SC: Subcutaneous administration

> Does the Healthcare Common Procedure Coding System include codes for pediatric vaccines? Not typically. Most codes for vaccines are found in *Current Procedural Terminology*.

VAR: Various routes of administration (used for drugs that are commonly administered into joints, cavities, tissues, or topical applications, in addition to other parenteral administrations)

> ### Billing for Drug Administration
>
> Note that inclusion of terms such as *injection* in the description of drugs references only how the drug was administered and does not preclude billing a *Current Procedural Terminology* code for the administration.

These abbreviations are important to accurate code selection from the Table of Drugs. Note that inclusion of terms such as *injection* in the description of drugs references only how the drug was administered and does not preclude billing a *CPT* code for the administration.

Table 4-3 shows an excerpt from the Table of Drugs listing for dexamethasone products. Note the cross-references from name brand Decadron and Decadron-LA to the generic listings. For each generic drug name, there are listings of

- Units—the smallest amount of the medication that equals 1 unit of service on your claim
- The required method of administration for the code
- The code for each listing

It is very important to find the correct drug and correct method of administration to arrive at the correct code. Once at the correct drug and route of administration, the correct number of units to report is based on the amount administered divided by the HCPCS unit.

> ### Determine HCPCS Units for Drugs
>
> The correct number of units to report is based on the amount administered divided by the Healthcare Common Procedure Coding System unit.

Example

You administer a single injection of ceftriaxone sodium 600 mg. You select code J0696 (injection, ceftriaxone sodium, per 250 mg).

To report the medication, you divide the 600 mg administered by the 250 mg in the HCPCS code descriptor and get 2.4 units. Medicare allows rounding up to bill 3 units, but other health plans may require reporting the exact 2.4 units. You separately report the appropriate *CPT* code for the drug administration.

Note that some codes describe medications that are administered by a single method.

- Dexamethasone, concentrated form (INH)
- Dexamethasone, intravitreal implant (OTH)
- Dexamethasone, oral (ORAL)

However, code **J1100** represents dexamethasone sodium phosphate when provided by intramuscular, intravenous, or other method of administration.

- Dexamethasone sodium phosphate (IM, IV, OTH)

Most drug codes listed in HCPCS are listed once with the lowest common denominator in which they are supplied. For example, Rocephin (ceftriaxone sodium) is available as 250 mg, 500 mg, 1 g, and 2 g. However, in the HCPCS code set there is only one code (**J0696**) "per 250 mg." One unit is reported for each 250 mg provided.

Table 4-3. Excerpt From HCPCS Table of Drugs			
Name	Units	Method	Code
Decadron Phosphate, see Dexamethasone sodium phosphate			
Decadron, see Dexamethasone sodium phosphate			
Decadron-LA, see Dexamethasone acetate			
Dexamethasone, concentrated form	per mg	INH	**J7637**
Dexamethasone, unit form	per mg	INH	**J7638**
Dexamethasone, intravitreal implant	0.1 mg	OTH	**J7312**
Dexamethasone, oral	0.25 mg	ORAL	**J8540**
Dexamethasone acetate	1 mg	IM	**J1094**
Dexamethasone sodium phosphate	1 mg	IM, IV, OTH	**J1100**
Dexasone, see Dexamethasone sodium phosphate			

Abbreviations: HCPCS, Healthcare Common Procedure Coding System; IM, intramuscular; INH, inhaled solution; IV, intravenous; ORAL, orally; OTH, other routes of administration.

HCPCS Coding Instructions

The most prominent instruction in the HCPCS manual is as follows:

> Questions regarding coding and billing guidance should be submitted to the insurer in whose jurisdiction a claim would be filed. For private sector health insurance systems, please contact the individual private insurance entity. For Medicaid systems, please contact the Medicaid Agency in the state in which the claim is being filed. For Medicare, contact the Medicare contractor.

Simply put, the health plan determines the coverage and payment guidelines for HCPCS codes. For pediatricians, this means that support staff in pediatric offices and facilities must maintain an awareness of payer guidelines for HCPCS code use.

- Many health plans and/or their administrative contractors publish payment policies and/or claim edits online to support correct coding.

- Payment policies are subject to change and should be monitored by administrative staff.

To see examples of payment policies, perform an internet search using "reimbursement policy <insert your 'state'> injections." (Using quotation marks before and after the state should limit results to policies for your state.) Policies often address whether or not supplies such as needles or tubing are separately reported, instructions for reporting drug codes, and billing for other services on the same date.

National Drug Codes (NDCs)

Medicaid plans and some other health plans may require a National Drug Code (NDC) on claims for drugs in addition to the appropriate HCPCS code to specifically identify the product administered. **Table 4-4** provides an overview of NDC uses and effective dates. See examples of NDCs in **Table 4-5**.

Table 4-4. National Drug Codes (NDCs) Overview	
Used to Report	**Effective Date**
Specific information on the labeler (drug company), drug product, and packaging	Updated daily as indicated for each new drug supplier, product, or packaging

National Drug Codes are maintained by the US Food and Drug Administration, which assigns the first 5 digits (*labeler identification*) of the NDC to the manufacturer, repackager, or distributor (the *labeler*) of a drug product. The labeler assigns the remaining digits to indicate the specific strength, dosage form (eg, tablet, liquid), and formulation of a drug and the packaging size or type. The NDC for a drug/vaccine may change as often as a labeler changes formulation or packaging.

- National Drug Codes may be entered into the patient record and/or added to billing information by the individual administering the drug.

- Many drugs have multiple NDCs based on how the drug is supplied (eg, single-dose vial, multiple-dose vial).

- Clinical and administrative staff must develop a process for capturing accurate NDCs for all drugs supplied in a practice.

- As shown in **Figure 4-1**, NDCs on drug products are 10-digit numbers. National Drug Code units on claims must be submitted in Health Insurance Portability and Accountability Act–compliant 11-digit format using a 5-4-2 format (ie, 5 digits, followed by 4 digits, followed by 2 digits). Examples of conversion to the 5-4-2 format are shown in **Table 4-5**.

- It is important to verify each payer's requirements for NDC reporting. A payer may require either of the following:

  > The NDC that is provided on the outer packaging when a vaccine or other drug is supplied in bulk packages

  > The NDC from the vial that was administered

Figure 4-1. National Drug Code on Drug Label

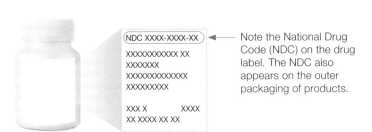

Note the National Drug Code (NDC) on the drug label. The NDC also appears on the outer packaging of products.

Table 4-5. National Drug Code Format Examples

Product	10-digit NDC Formats	11-digit NDC Formats (Added 0 [zero] is underscored.)
RotaTeq 2-mL single-dose tube, package of 20	**0006-4047-20** (4-4-2)	**00006-4047-20** (5-4-2)
Fluzone Quadrivalent 0.25-mL prefilled single-dose syringe, package of 10	**49281-517-25** (5-3-2)	**49281-0517-25** (5-4-2)
Synagis 0.5-mL in 1 vial, single dose	**60574-4114-1** (5-4-1)	**60574-4114-01** (5-4-2)

Abbreviation: NDC, National Drug Code.

NDC Units of Service

Units of service for NDCs are often not the same as units of service for HCPCS codes. National Drug Codes appear on the same service line of a claim as the HCPCS code in the shaded row above fields 24A through 24G. See the 1500 claim form example in **Figure 4-2** for examples of how NDCs and units are reported on claims.

Figure 4-2. Example of National Drug Code Reporting on 1500 Claim Form

Abbreviations: DTaP, diphtheria, tetanus, acellular pertussis; E/M, evaluation and management; Hib, *Haemophilus influenzae* type b; IPV, inactivated poliovirus; PCV13, pneumococcal conjugate; RV5, rotavirus.

Note that an identifier (N4) precedes the NDCs on the claim.

For most payers, NDC units are reported as grams (GR), milligrams (ME), milliliters (ML), or units (UN). In **Figure 4-2**, units of service in milliliters (ML) follow the NDCs. (In contrast, *CPT* codes for vaccines are reported with 1 unit per vaccine product in field 24G.)

Coding Keys

- **There are multiple levels of Healthcare Common Procedure Coding System (HCPCS) codes.** *Current Procedural Terminology* (*CPT®*) codes are also referred to as Level I HCPCS codes. Level II HCPCS codes are used to report the following items not described by *CPT* codes:
    - > Supplies
    - > Medications
    - > Services (when a *CPT* code does not describe the service as covered by health plan benefits)
- **HCPCS or *CPT*?** Choose a HCPCS code when no *CPT* code adequately describes the service or as required by a specific health plan. When both a *CPT* and HCPCS Level II code have the same descriptor, use the *CPT* code unless a health plan requires the HCPCS code.
- **How HCPCS code updates happen:** The Centers for Medicare & Medicaid Services (CMS) maintains the HCPCS code set, and codes can be added, changed, or discontinued on a quarterly basis. Newly established temporary codes are usually implemented within 90 days of publication; otherwise, HCPCS codes are updated annually on January 1.
- **How can you identify a HCPCS code?** HCPCS codes are alphanumeric and composed of a letter followed by 4 numbers. The letter serves as a signal to the type of service listed under the code (eg, drugs are listed under **J**; pathology and laboratory services are under **P**; diagnostic radiology services are under **R**).
- **Just like *CPT* codes, HCPCS codes can incorporate modifiers.** HCPCS modifiers are 2 characters and may contain numbers or letters. They convey specific information not covered by code descriptions or *CPT* modifiers, such as right side (modifier **RT**) or upper left eyelid (**E1**).
- **Tips for navigating a HCPCS manual**
    - > For **supplies and services other than drugs**, start in the alphabetical index. Searchable electronic HCPCS manuals are often more user-friendly for locating codes.
    - > For **drugs**, reference the Table of Drugs, which includes brand and generic drug names, dose per unit billed, and route of administration, such as IA (intra-arterial administration) or SC (subcutaneous administration).
- **National Drug Codes (NDCs):** Some health plans, including Medicaid, may require an NDC on claims. The NDC is a 10-digit number that can be located on the drug label as well as its outer packaging. It is important to verify each payer's requirements for NDC reporting.

Resources

CLIA Test Categorization

- Waived test systems and analytes (www.accessdata.fda.gov/scripts/cdrh/cfdocs/ cfClia/analyteswaived.cfm)
- Centers for Medicare & Medicaid Services CLIA categorization (www.cms.hhs.gov/ CLIA)

HCPCS Codes

- American Hospital Association *Coding Clinic* (https://www.codingclinicadvisor.com)

National Drug Codes

- US Food and Drug Administration NDC Directory (www.fda.gov/drugs/drug-approvals-and-databases/national-drug-code-directory)

Coding Challenge

(Answers may be found in Appendix A.)

1. True or false? Healthcare Common Procedure Coding System (HCPCS) codes are composed of 5 numerical characters.

    a. True

    b. False

2. What information is included in the HCPCS Table of Drugs?

    a. Brand names of medications

    b. Generic names of medications

    c. Method of administration

    d. All of the above

3. Which of the following indicates the laterality of a procedure or service?

    a. Modifier **XE**

    b. Modifier **QW**

    c. HCPCS code

    d. Modifier **LT** or **RT**

4. How often are HCPCS code updates implemented?

    a. Annually, January 1

    b. Each January 1, with quarterly updates for temporary codes

    c. October 1

    d. As needed throughout the year

Chapter 5

Coding Assignment and Billing Processes

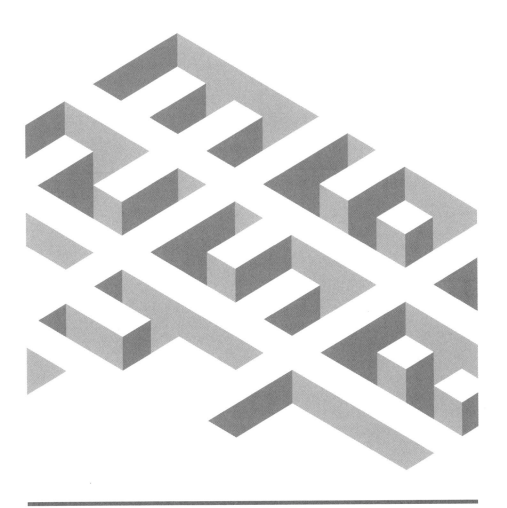

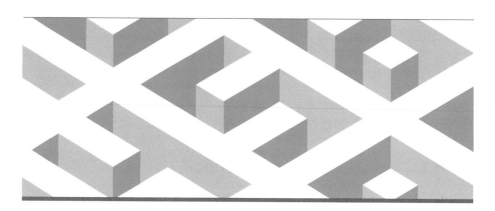

Codes Tell the Encounter Story

In chapters 1 through 4, we discussed why coding matters to pediatricians, characteristics of each code set (ie, *International Classification of Diseases, 10th Revision, Clinical Modification [ICD-10-CM]*; *Current Procedural Terminology (CPT®)*; Healthcare Common Procedure Coding System [HCPCS]; and National Drug Code [NDC]), how codes are found in each manual, and some key tips for reporting the codes. Once codes are selected, they must be appropriately placed on a claim form to tell the story of what took place in an encounter and why.

The codes submitted on a claim tell the story of what happened during a patient encounter based on what the pediatrician and other providers of care documented in the patient record. When codes are sufficient to describe what services were provided to a patient and why the services were needed, claims can be promptly considered for payment. An incomplete story causes a delay in payment.

Appropriate *ICD-10-CM* codes describe the reasons for services.

- Preventive care: **Z23**, encounter for immunization
- Exposure to infectious disease: **Z20.811**, contact with and (suspected) exposure to meningococcus
- Signs and symptoms: **R68.12**, fussy infant (baby)
- Diagnosed conditions: **J02.0**, streptococcal pharyngitis
- Medical history: **Z87.74**, personal history of (corrected) congenital malformations of heart and circulatory system
- Family medical history: **Z82.5**, family history of asthma and other chronic lower respiratory diseases

Correctly assigning and linking diagnosis codes to services and supplies on the claim provides a health plan with an indication of the reason that each service or supply was clinically indicated. See **Figure 5-1** for an illustration of how *ICD-10-CM* codes are linked to *CPT* or HCPCS codes on the service lines of a claim.

Most services can be distinctly described by procedure codes.

10120	Incision and removal of foreign body, subcutaneous tissues; simple
69200	Removal foreign body from external auditory canal; without general anesthesia
99238	Hospital discharge day management; 30 minutes or less
99291	Critical care, evaluation and management of the critically ill or critically injured patient; first 30-74 minutes

When indicated, modifiers should be appended to codes to tell more about a service.

25	Significant, separately identifiable evaluation and management service by the same physician or other qualified health care professional on the same day of the procedure or other service
50	Bilateral procedure
F4	Left hand, fifth digit

Additional codes can be added to describe medications and supplies.

Q4011	Cast supplies, short arm cast, pediatric [0-10 years], plaster
99070	Supplies and materials (This code requires additional description on the claim form.)
J2357	Injection, omalizumab, 5 mg (Describes only the generic drug and dosage. One unit is reported for each 5 mg.)
50242-0214-01	Omalizumab 75 mg/0.5mL (The 11-digit NDC code conveys the exact product provided. One unit is reported for each 0.5-mL prefilled syringe.)

Claims also contain narrative fields where additional explanations (eg, reasons a service was more or less intense than typical) may be provided, when indicated.

Figure 5-1. Example of Diagnosis Linking

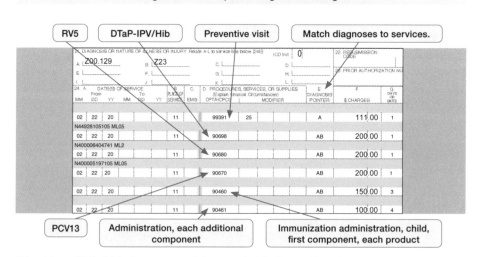

Abbreviations: DTaP, diphtheria, tetanus, acellular pertussis; Hib, *Haemophilus influenzae* type b; IPV, inactived poliovirus; PCV13, pneumococcal conjugate; RV5, rotavirus.

Figure 5-2 illustrates how each code provides a part of the story of what services were provided and why

Figure 5-2. The Encounter Story Through Codes

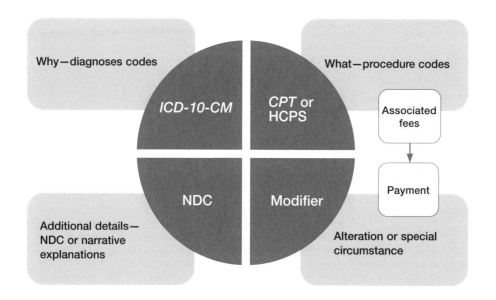

Abbreviations: *CPT, Current Procedural Terminology;* HCPCS, Healthcare Common Procedure Coding System; *ICD-10-CM, International Classification of Diseases, 10th Revision, Clinical Modification;* NDC, National Drug Code.

A single encounter may include multiple diagnosis and procedure codes. For instance, a child is seen for a well-child visit (reported as a preventive medicine evaluation and management [E/M] service). You might report a single diagnosis code indicating a routine health examination…

Z00.129	Encounter for routine child health examination without abnormal findings

…and a single procedure code.

99384	Initial comprehensive preventive medicine evaluation and management of an individual including an age and gender appropriate history, examination, counseling/anticipatory guidance/risk factor reduction interventions, and the ordering of laboratory/diagnostic procedures, new patient; adolescent (age 12 through 17 years)

However, you might also order an influenza immunization and perform routine developmental screening. You assign codes for each diagnosis or reason for a service.

Z00.129	Encounter for routine child health examination without abnormal findings
Z23	Encounter for immunization
Z13.42	Encounter for screening for global developmental delays (milestones)

You also assign procedure codes for each service provided and any billable supplies (eg, vaccine or toxoid administered). For example

99382 25	Initial comprehensive preventive medicine evaluation and management of an individual including an age and gender appropriate history, examination, counseling/anticipatory guidance/risk factor reduction interventions, and the ordering of laboratory/diagnostic procedures, new patient; early childhood (age 1 through 4 years)
96110	Developmental screening (eg, developmental milestone survey, speech and language delay screen), with scoring and documentation, per standardized instrument
90460	Immunization administration through 18 years of age via any route of administration, with counseling by physician or other qualified health care professional; first or only component of each vaccine or toxoid administered
90655	Influenza virus vaccine, trivalent (IIV3), split virus, preservative free, 0.25 mL dosage, for intramuscular use

Pediatricians should follow each code set's guidelines for assignment of multiple codes. Modifiers, such as modifier **25** in the previous example, are often required to provide additional information about services provided. Modifier use is discussed in Chapter 3.

Telling Your Story on a Claim

When codes have been assigned to the documented services provided for an encounter, charges for the encounter are sent to health plans via electronic claim submission (most commonly) or on a paper 1500 claim form.

Most electronic billing systems are configured to collect and appropriately populate electronic or paper claims.

- Understanding the information required for claims processing by a health plan is helpful in using these electronic systems and claims adjudication processes to their full potential.
- Clean claims, those that contain all information necessary for the health plan to determine benefit payments, are subject to prompt payment regulations in most states. However, claims that do not contain all information necessary for processing are often delayed or denied.

The National Uniform Claim Committee (NUCC) provides an instruction manual for completing the 1500 claim form (www.nucc.org/index.php/1500-claim-form-mainmenu-35/1500-instructions-mainmenu-42). The single-page claim form contains key information required to determine benefit eligibility of the patient and coverage of the services provided. This includes

- Identification of the patient/insured and any other insurance that may cover the services (items 1–13)

- Accident or pregnancy information, when applicable (items 14–16)

- Referring providers, when applicable (items 17–17b)

- Diagnosis codes (21)

> ### Place of Service Codes
>
> Two-digit codes identify where a service was provided. These are typically entered into an electronic billing system once for each location where services are provided and automatically applied to each claim based on the location selected at charge entry.

- Dates, place of service codes, procedure codes, modifiers, link to supporting diagnosis code(s), units of service, and identification of pediatrician or other health care professional (items 24A–J, 1–6, and 28 and 29)

- Patient account number assigned by practice (item 26)

- Practice information (items 25, 31, and 33)

- Service facility (eg, hospital) location (item 32)

The 1500 claim form (**Figure 5-3**) illustrates the information that is included on an electronic or a paper claim. (See Appendix B, Glossary of Common Coding Acronyms, as needed.) Although only 6 service lines are included on a 1500 claim form, multiple forms may be used when more than 6 services are billed. Electronic claims may contain as many as 50 service lines. Up to 4 diagnosis codes may be linked to each service line.

An Overview of the Billing Process

Pediatricians are not typically directly involved with the billing and collection activities of their practice. However, knowledge of the process is beneficial to understanding the importance of working with and providing oversight (when indicated) to knowledgeable front desk and billing office staff members.

Despite the benefits of standardization, a chain of events from patient scheduling to posting of payments must be well coordinated to achieve accurate payment for pediatric services. Pediatricians can benefit from understanding the basic steps in the process of getting paid, although many steps take place before and after the patient visit and are taken by nonclinical staff who may work for or on contract with the pediatric practice.

Billing begins at the time appointments are scheduled and patient insurance information is collected and verified to provide benefits for a pediatrician's services (eg, in-network status). Collection and verification of current patient and health plan information is necessary at each encounter.

Figure 5-3. 1500 Claim Form

Example 1500 Claim Form

ABC Health Plan
123 Money St.
Anywhere, AK 00000

CARRIER

HEALTH INSURANCE CLAIM FORM

APPROVED BY NATIONAL UNIFORM CLAIM COMMITTEE (NUCC) 02/12

PICA | PICA

PATIENT AND INSURED INFORMATION

1. MEDICARE (Medicare#) ☐ MEDICAID (Medicaid#) ☒ TRICARE (ID#/DoD#) ☐ CHAMPVA (Member ID#) ☐ GROUP HEALTH PLAN (ID#) ☐ FECA BLK LUNG (ID#) ☐ OTHER (ID#) ☐		1a. INSURED'S I.D. NUMBER (For Program in Item 1) 123456789
2. PATIENT'S NAME (Last Name, First Name, Middle Initial) Smith, Boy	3. PATIENT'S BIRTH DATE MM DD YY 11 22 2018 SEX M ☒ F ☐	4. INSURED'S NAME (Last Name, First Name, Middle Initial) Smith, Momma
5. PATIENT'S ADDRESS (No., Street) 123 Main St.	6. PATIENT RELATIONSHIP TO INSURED Self ☒ Spouse ☐ Child ☐ Other ☐	7. INSURED'S ADDRESS (No., Street)
CITY Anywhere STATE KS	8. RESERVED FOR NUCC USE	CITY STATE
ZIP CODE 12345 TELEPHONE (Include Area Code) (555) 5555555		ZIP CODE TELEPHONE (Include Area Code) ( )
9. OTHER INSURED'S NAME (Last Name, First Name, Middle Initial) Smith, Poppa	10. IS PATIENT'S CONDITION RELATED TO:	11. INSURED'S POLICY GROUP OR FECA NUMBER 98765432102
a. OTHER INSURED'S POLICY OR GROUP NUMBER 45612378900	a. EMPLOYMENT? (Current or Previous) ☐ YES ☒ NO	a. INSURED'S DATE OF BIRTH MM DD YY 01 01 1992 SEX M ☐ F ☒
b. RESERVED FOR NUCC USE	b. AUTO ACCIDENT? PLACE (State) ☐ YES ☒ NO	b. OTHER CLAIM ID (Designated by NUCC)
c. RESERVED FOR NUCC USE	c. OTHER ACCIDENT? ☐ YES ☒ NO	c. INSURANCE PLAN NAME OR PROGRAM NAME Good Health Plan
d. INSURANCE PLAN NAME OR PROGRAM NAME Another Good Plan	10d. CLAIM CODES (Designated by NUCC)	d. IS THERE ANOTHER HEALTH BENEFIT PLAN? ☒ YES ☐ NO *If yes*, complete items 9, 9a, and 9d.

READ BACK OF FORM BEFORE COMPLETING & SIGNING THIS FORM.

12. PATIENT'S OR AUTHORIZED PERSON'S SIGNATURE I authorize the release of any medical or other information necessary to process this claim. I also request payment of government benefits either to myself or to the party who accepts assignment below.

SIGNED Signature on file DATE 02/22/2019

13. INSURED'S OR AUTHORIZED PERSON'S SIGNATURE I authorize payment of medical benefits to the undersigned physician or supplier for services described below.

SIGNED Signature on file

PHYSICIAN OR SUPPLIER INFORMATION

14. DATE OF CURRENT ILLNESS, INJURY, or PREGNANCY (LMP)
MM | DD | YY   QUAL.

15. OTHER DATE   MM | DD | YY   QUAL.

16. DATES PATIENT UNABLE TO WORK IN CURRENT OCCUPATION
FROM MM | DD | YY   TO MM | DD | YY

17. NAME OF REFERRING PROVIDER OR OTHER SOURCE
17a.
17b. NPI

18. HOSPITALIZATION DATES RELATED TO CURRENT SERVICES
FROM MM | DD | YY   TO MM | DD | YY

19. ADDITIONAL CLAIM INFORMATION (Designated by NUCC)

20. OUTSIDE LAB?   ☐ YES ☐ NO $ CHARGES

21. DIAGNOSIS OR NATURE OF ILLNESS OR INJURY Relate A-L to service line below (24E)   ICD Ind. | 0 |
A. Z00.129   B. Z23   C. | | D. |
E. | | F. | | G. | | H. |
I. | | J. | | K. | | L. |

22. RESUBMISSION CODE | ORIGINAL REF NO

23. PRIOR AUTHORIZATION NUMBER

24. A. DATE(S) OF SERVICE From MM DD YY To MM DD YY	B. PLACE OF SERVICE	C. EMG	D. PROCEDURES, SERVICES, OR SUPPLIES (Explain Unusual Circumstances) CPT/HCPCS	MODIFIER	E. DIAGNOSIS POINTER	F. $ CHARGES	G. DAYS OR UNITS	H. EPSDT Family Plan	I. ID QUAL.	J. RENDERING PROVIDER ID. #
02 22 20	11		99391	25	A	111|00	1		NPI	1234567890
N449281051725 ML05										
02 22 20	11		90698		AB	200|00	1		NPI	1234567890
N400006404741 ML2										
02 22 20	11		90680		AB	200|00	1		NPI	1234567890
N400005197105 ML05										
02 22 20	11		90670		AB	200|00	1		NPI	1234567890
02 22 20	11		90460		AB	150|00	3		NPI	1234567890
02 22 20	11		90461		AB	100|00	4		NPI	1234567890

25. FEDERAL TAX I.D. NUMBER   SSN ☐ EIN ☒
12-4567897

26. PATIENT'S ACCOUNT NO
11111

27. ACCEPT ASSIGNMENT? (For govt. claims, see back)
☒ YES ☐ NO

28. TOTAL CHARGE $ 961\|00

29. AMOUNT PAID $

30. Rsvd for NUCC Use

31. SIGNATURE OF PHYSICIAN OR SUPPLIER INCLUDING DEGREES OR CREDENTIALS
(I certify that the statements on the reverse apply to this bill and are made a part thereof.)
Signature on file
SIGNED   DATE 02/23/2019

32. SERVICE FACILITY LOCATION INFORMATION
Pediatric Practice
111 Some St
Anywhere, US 99999
a. | b.

33. BILLING PROVIDER INFO & PH # (555) 555-5555
Pediatric Practice
111 Some St
Anywhere, US 99999
a. 0123456789 | b.

NUCC Instruction Manual available at www.nucc.org   PLEASE PRINT OR TYPE   APPROVED OMB-0938-1197 FORM 1500 (02-12)

Billing office staff members or a billing service is responsible for many steps to correct payment.

- Preparing and submitting initial claims
- Following up on unpaid claims in a timely manner
- Maintaining awareness of timely filing policies of payers to avoid denials caused by delayed filing of claims
- Holding payers accountable for meeting agreed-on or state-mandated time for payment of clean claims
- Correcting and resubmitting claims when rejected or denied
- Appealing wrongly denied claims
- Posting payments and adjustments (amount of charge above contractually agreed-on payment)
- Posting write-offs approved by practice administrators (eg, bad debt, charitable care)
- Billing for and following up on amounts due from patient/caregiver
- Advising practice administrators of necessary refunds (eg, patient overpayment, duplicate health plan payment)

Figure 5-4 shows steps from patient scheduling to payment and account reconciliation.

Figure 5-4. Billing Cycle for Health Care Professional Services

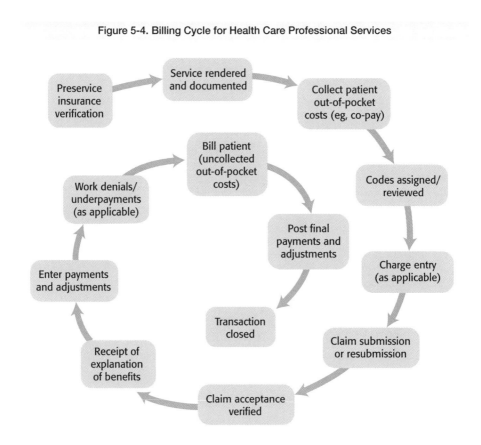

Reconciling Charges

An important process in the billing cycle is verification that the practice has received the correct payment from health plans and the patient's caregivers, as applicable. Claims may be delayed for additional information, denied correctly or in error, or paid at a rate different than the contractually agreed-on amounts. Billing staff members must have processes in place to track and follow up with health plans on unpaid or incorrectly paid claims. Amounts billed to patients must align with health plan remittance advice.

Write-offs and Adjustments

Pediatricians typically contract to participate in health plan networks and, in doing so, agree to accept the health plan's fee schedule (allowable amount to be paid per service) and payment policies. This creates complexity in the billing and payment of services.

Example

You provide an office visit to a new patient and report code 99203 with a charge of $180 and a laboratory test charge of $40. The remittance advice from the health plan might show the following:

Tip: Collecting Patient Balances

Co-payments should be collected at the time of service. It is also possible to use electronic verification of benefits to identify the amount of deductible not met and collect that portion of the allowed amount at the time of service, when applicable.

Example Remittance Advice							
Billed Amount	Allowed Amount	Contractual Adjustment	Deductible	Co-payment	Coinsurance	Amount Paid	Patient Responsibility
$180	$119	$61	$0	$20	$0	$99	$20
$40	$22	$18	$22	$0	$0	$0	$22
$220	$141	$79	$22	$20	$0	$99	$42

Abbreviation: NDC, National Drug Code.

Based on the contracted fee schedule, you must accept $141 as payment in full for the services billed at $220.

- $79 is adjusted off the account balance.

- The health plan paid $99 of the $141 allowed amount.

- $42 was applied to the patient's deductible and co-payment (payable by the patient's parent/caregiver).

Terms used on remittance advices can be confusing to patients and those new to health insurance terminology. These include

- *Contractual adjustment:* The amount you must adjust off your charge because of your contractual agreement with the health plan

- *Deductible:* A designated amount a patient pays out of pocket before the health plan pays

- *Co-payment:* An out-of-pocket cost to the patient; usually applicable to office and emergency department visits

- *Coinsurance:* A percentage of allowed charges that the patient must pay out of pocket (usually capped at a specific amount)

Although the patient has coverage for the service under the health plan, the deductible and co-payment totaling $42 are the patient or caregiver's responsibility. If the patient has a secondary insurance, the remaining balance would be billed to that plan with a copy of the primary plan's remittance. If not, a bill for the unpaid balance would be sent to the patient or caregiver. Pediatric practices must be careful to not bill patients for amounts that must be adjusted off due to contractual obligation.

Patient Billing Concerns

At times, parents and other caregivers will speak directly with pediatricians about their bill and/or ability to pay for recommended or received services. It is best to establish a practice policy addressing how these conversations will be handled (eg, referral to billing manager). Practices that establish policies and procedures for responding to billing concerns and/or requests for discounts (eg, prompt payment, financial hardship) can more effectively respond.

Patient Discounts

Pediatricians must not advertise discounting of patient deductibles or other out-of-pocket costs associated with health plan policies or government-funded health coverage. Federal and state regulations and health plan contracts typically prohibit discounts for reasons other than substantiated financial hardship. Discounts for prompt payment of self-pay or out-of-pocket costs above certain amounts may also be acceptable.

Policies about billing communications and patient discounts must align with health plan contracts and federal and state regulations (eg, avoid improper incentives for patients to receive services or supplies). Policies form a basis on which procedures are developed and implemented.

Standardized procedures create efficiency and help avoid risks of noncompliance with contractual obligation or regulatory requirements.

The American Academy of Pediatrics has template letters (in Word) related to payment, available at https://www.aap.org/en-us/professional-resources/practice-transformation/managing-patients/Pages/template-letters-sample-policies.aspx, that pediatric practices can customize on topics such as

- Notification of practice financial policies
- Families without health insurance
- Response to questions about bills
- Practices no longer contracting with health plans
- Practice policies for patients awaiting Medicaid approval

Pediatricians may also receive complaints about how billing and/or communications about billing are handled by practice staff members. Again, policies and procedures should guide a pediatrician's response (eg, acknowledgment of the parent/caregiver's concern and hand off to appropriate billing office or practice manager).

Patient and parent/caregiver satisfaction with quality medical care may be reduced by bad experiences with the billing office/service. All billing office staff members should be considered patient facing and undergo routine customer service and compliance training. Practice managers must maintain awareness of and effectively manage the practice's communications about unpaid claims and patient balances.

Coding Keys

- **Keep your claims clean.** Clean claims contain all the information necessary for a health plan to determine benefit payments and provide prompt payment. Claims that do not contain all necessary information are often delayed or denied.

- **The 1500 claim form:** While most claims are sent to health plans electronically, some are still submitted using the paper 1500 claim form. The National Uniform Claim Committee (NUCC) provides an instruction manual for completing the single-page form. The form contains key information required to determine benefit eligibility of the patient and coverage of the services provided.

- **Reconciling charges:** It's important to verify that a practice has received the correct payment from health plans and the patient's caregivers, as applicable. Billing staff members should establish a process to track and follow up with health plans on unpaid or incorrectly paid claims.

- **Navigating network payment amounts:** When pediatricians contract to participate in a health plan network, they agree to accept the health plan's fee schedule and payment policies. This can create confusion for billing staff and patients reviewing remittance advice. For example, if services would typically be billed at $220 but the health plan will only pay the allowed amount of $141, you must accept $141 as payment in full.

Resources

American Academy of Pediatrics

- Coding Hotline (www.aap.org/en-us/Pages/cu/Coding-Hotline-Request.aspx)
- Coding Webinars (www.aap.org/en-us/professional-resources/practice-transformation/getting-paid/Coding-at-the-AAP/Pages/AAP-Coding-Webinars.aspx)
- *AAP Pediatric Coding Newsletter*™ (http://coding.aap.org)
- Policy statement, "A New Era in Quality Measurement: The Development and Application of Quality Measures" (http://pediatrics.aappublications.org/content/139/1/e20163442)
- Payment-related template letters (https://www.aap.org/en-us/professional-resources/practice-transformation/managing-patients/Pages/template-letters-sample-policies.aspx)

Claims Processing

- Improving Claims Processing and Payment: A Self-Assessment Tool for Physicians/Providers (www.aap.org/en-us/Documents/ImprovingClaimsProcessing.pdf)
- Claim adjustment reason code and remittance advice remark code descriptions (www.wpc-edi.com/reference)
- National Uniform Claim Committee (www.nucc.org/index.php/1500-claim-form-mainmenu-35/1500-instructions-mainmenu-42)

Current Procedural Terminology

- American Academy of Pediatrics *Coding for Pediatrics* (www.aap.org/cfp)
- American Medical Association *CPT* general information (www.ama-assn.org/practice-management/cpt-current-procedural-terminology)
- *CPT* Category II codes and alphabetical clinical topics listing (www.ama-assn.org/practice-management/cpt-category-ii-codes)

ICD-10-CM Code Files and Guidelines

- American Academy of Pediatrics *Pediatric ICD-10-CM: A Manual for Provider-Based Coding* (https://shop.aap.org)
- National Center for Health Statistics *ICD-10-CM* (www.cdc.gov/nchs/icd/icd10cm.htm)

Quality Measures

- Quality measurement at the AAP (www.aap.org/en-us/professional-resources/quality-improvement/Pages/quality-measurement.aspx)
- National Committee for Quality Assurance (www.ncqa.org)
- Physician Consortium for Performance Improvement (www.thepcpi.org)

Place of Service Codes

- Place of service code set (www.cms.gov/Medicare/Coding/place-of-service-codes/Place_of_Service_Code_Set.html)

Coding Challenge

(Answers may be found in Appendix A.)

1. Correctly assigning and linking diagnosis codes to services and supplies on a claim provides a health plan with what information?

    a. The reason that each service or supply was clinically indicated

    b. What services were provided

    c. Alterations or special circumstances in how a service was provided

    d. All of the above

2. True or false? You must assign only one diagnosis per claim line.

    a. True

    b. False

3. What do you call the amount you must adjust off your charge because of your contractual agreement with the health plan?

    a. Deductible

    b. Patient balance

    c. Contractual adjustment

    d. Modifier

4. What is a *clean claim*?

    a. A claim with only one service line

    b. A claim containing all information necessary for the health plan to determine benefit payments

    c. A claim that is filed on the same date the service was provided

    d. A claim that contains up to 6 service lines

Chapter 6

Health Plan Policies and Coding Compliance

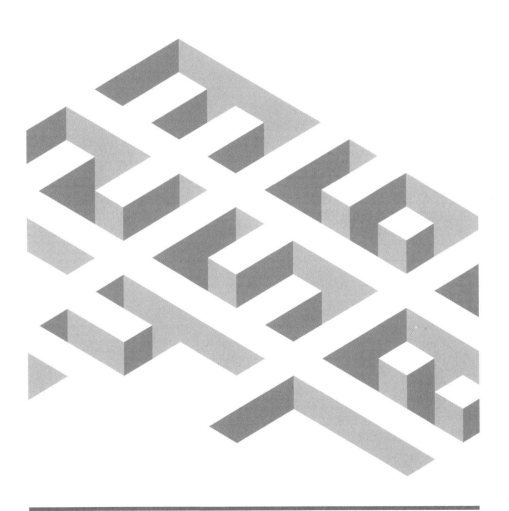

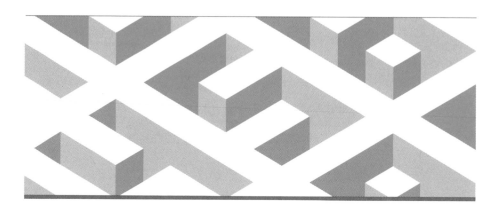

Covered Services

As previously noted, most pediatric services are billed to health plans before or in lieu of billing to the patient or caregiver.

- Pediatricians typically sign participation agreements or contracts with these health plans that require billing and coding in compliance with the health plan policies.
- Health plans limit payment of benefits to only those services covered by the plan and provided in compliance with the plan or state Medicaid policies and procedures.

Medical Necessity

One concept included in nearly all health plan contracts is that, aside from recommended preventive services, payment will be made only for services that are "medically necessary."

> **Health care interventions are evidence based, evidence informed, or based on consensus advisory opinion and are recommended by recognized health care professionals, such as the American Academy of Pediatrics, to promote optimal growth and development in a child and to prevent, detect, diagnose, treat, ameliorate, or palliate the effects of physical, genetic, congenital, developmental, behavioral, or mental conditions, injuries, or disabilities.**

Example

A health plan usually will not cover cosmetic procedures (eg, otoplasty [ear pinning]) that are not also therapeutic or to improve function of a body part.

Medical necessity is a mechanism that gives legal authority to a health plan to limit the provision of covered benefits to an enrollee. Medicare policy instructs auditors that medically necessary services are

- Safe and effective
- Not experimental or investigational
- Appropriate, including the duration and frequency in terms of whether the service or item is
  - > Furnished in accordance with accepted standards of medical practice for the diagnosis or treatment of the beneficiary's condition or to improve the function of a malformed body member
  - > Furnished in a setting appropriate to the beneficiary's medical needs and condition

> Ordered and furnished by qualified personnel

> One that meets, but does not exceed, the beneficiary's medical need

Services deemed not medically necessary may be billable to the patient or caregiver when allowed by the health plan contract. This typically requires a pediatrician to obtain a form completed and signed by the patient or caregiver, prior to receipt of services, documenting the service to be provided, the total cost of the service, and an agreement to pay out of pocket for services if denied because of medical necessity.

Coding Compliance

Just as patients put enormous trust in physicians, so do payers. Medicare, Medicaid, other federal health care programs, and private payers rely on physicians' medical judgment to treat patients with appropriate services.

They depend on physicians to submit accurate and truthful claims for the services provided to their enrollees. And most physicians intend to do just that. However, the process is made more difficult by the complex and dynamic nature of payer coding and billing procedures, which, despite efforts to standardize, persist from carrier to carrier, policy to policy, state to state, and month to month.

While health plan edits may catch most coding and billing errors, pediatricians must incorporate coding compliance education and monitoring into their practice to avoid inadvertent abusive coding practices and/or lost revenue caused by inaccurate coding.

- Pediatric practices benefit from having compliance initiatives because they tighten billing and coding operations and can improve documentation.

- Practices with written compliance programs report having better control on internal procedures, improved medical record documentation, and streamlined practice operations.

Pediatricians who take time to learn about and support compliant coding and billing practices not only benefit from more accurate payment but also avoid risks associated with erroneous coding, including

- Denied claims

- Underpayment or overpayment that requires reconciliation with a payer and/or patient

- Recoupment of amounts previously paid

- Potential violations of fraud and abuse regulations and associated penalties

Medicare, state Medicaid programs, and health plans will audit claims as well as monitor the levels of evaluation and management (E/M) services (eg, office visits) reported by pediatricians. With coding education and a structured compliance program, pediatricians can be prepared to appropriately document and defend the codes reported for their services.

Pediatricians who do not take time to learn about and support compliant coding and billing practices may lose significant revenue caused by

- Unbilled or under-coded charges
- Repayment demands from health plans
- Time and resources spent complying with audits and investigations
- Charges of abusive billing practice and/or fraud

Do not take risks with coding and billing. Not only are these the means of having a practice with reliable income, but documented efforts at compliant coding and billing are a protection against accusations of abusive billing practices and/or fraud.

One case example of noncompliant coding and billing in recent years was a New Jersey pediatrician found guilty of 48 counts of health care claims fraud and 1 count of Medicaid fraud for billing for more than 24 hours of services per day on 48 days despite her office being open only 3 days per week for 8 hours per day. The pediatrician was sentenced to 3 years in prison.

Protecting your practice and yourself while sustaining a profitable practice depends on complete documentation of services and accurate coding and billing.

Code Edits

Health plans use many methods to ensure that benefits are paid only for medically necessary and/or preventive services that are included in the plan's benefits. Code edits are used to automate the claims adjudication process. Based on edits, electronic programs allow or deny charges for services reported on each claim.

The claims processing program is set up to recognize codes for services that may not be covered or for which payment is included in another service. The claims processing program also evaluates claims with relation to claims billed by other health care professionals on the same and/or different days of service.

- Edits for some codes are set to result in denial of associated charges because the plan does not cover the service described by the code or the code is no longer valid. Obtaining a full list of covered codes from each of your payers is essential to avoid unexpected denial of claims.

Most health plans consider physicians of the same group practice and specialty as one physician when each provides services to the same patient on the same date.

- Many codes are subject to payment edits that can result in denial if the service represented by the code is considered a component of another code billed for the same patient by the same physician (or a physician of the same group practice and same specialty) on the same date of service. Some services are subject to inclusion in the payment for a procedure for a specified time or global period (usually 0, 10, or 90 days following the day of a procedural service). Charges for visits provided during the global period are denied. (See more in the Global Period Edits section later in this chapter.)

- Some codes are subject to limitations on how many units may be billed on the same date or within a specified period based on health plan policies. (See the Medically Unlikely Edits section later in this chapter.)

- Certain services may be eligible for benefit payment only when provided to treat or manage certain conditions. Combinations of procedure and diagnosis codes are used to determine if the service reported is eligible for benefit payment. Health plans typically define these in national and local coverage determinations that are often published on the plan's website.

Examples

You provide a patient with an immunization.

The code for the vaccine is erroneously reported with 2 units instead of 1. A claims adjudication system may allow payment of the fee schedule amount for 1 unit (1 vaccine product) and deny the remainder of the charge.

You repair a wound on a patient's foot and tell the patient to return in 7 days for suture removal.

The code for the repair is assigned a 10-day global period (ie, payment for the code includes the procedure and all related services for 10 days after the date of the procedure). You bill an office visit (eg, **99213**) for the visit to remove sutures that takes place within the global period. The charge is denied due to inclusion in the global period.

National Correct Coding Initiative Edits

National Correct Coding Initiative (NCCI) edits are sets of claims processing edits used by Medicare and Medicaid programs. The Centers for Medicare & Medicaid Services (CMS) developed the NCCI to promote national correct coding methodologies and to control improper coding leading to inappropriate payment in Medicare Part B claims. Later, legislation required the CMS to expand the NCCI to the Medicaid program to reduce improper coding and erroneous claims payment.

The NCCI is also now used by many private and government-funded health plans (eg, Tricare military health system). Individual health plans may adopt Medicare or Medicaid code edits (in full or in part) or may create their own code edits.

- The CMS releases the Medicare NCCI edits free of charge on its website (www.cms. gov/NationalCorrectCodInitEd/NCCIEP/list.asp).

- Medicaid NCCI files are published separately free of charge at www.medicaid.gov/ medicaid/program-integrity/ncci/edit-files/index.html.

- Although many Medicare and Medicaid edits are the same, there are variations.

- The CMS publishes manuals for Medicare and Medicaid NCCI edits to help users understand the purpose and intent of the edits. See the websites for Medicare and Medicaid NCCI edits for the corresponding manuals.

There are 2 types of NCCI edits.

- Procedure-to-procedure (PTP) edits pair codes to prevent improper payment when incorrect code combinations are reported (eg, codes for tonsillectomy and adenoidectomy are paired because another code for the combined procedures should be reported).

- Medically Unlikely Edits (MUEs) limit the number of units of service allowed on one date. This helps to eliminate inaccurate payment caused by errors in the number of units reported (eg, 100 units is billed when 10 were provided).

Procedure-to-Procedure Edits

Procedure-to-procedure edits preclude billing of paired codes for services to a single patient by the same physician on the same date of service.

- These code edits appear in column 1 and column 2 of the same row in a table of NCCI edits.

- Modifier indicators **0** or **1** advise whether use of a clinically indicated modifier will result in override of the code pair edit.

  > **0**: The code pair cannot be billed under any circumstances.

  > **1**: An NCCI-associated modifier will override the edit (see the Modifiers section later in this chapter).

- Effective dates and, when applicable, deletion dates are included for all code pairs.

Table 6-1 provides examples of codes paired in column 1 and column 2 and a modifier indicator for each. Below each row with a pair of codes is an explanation of how the edit affects payment.

Table 6-1. Examples of Medicaid National Correct Coding Initiative Procedure-to-Procedure Edits			
Column 1	Column 2	Modifier Indicator	Effective Date
94060 Bronchodilation responsiveness, spirometry as in **94010**, pre- and post-bronchodilator administration	**94010** Spirometry	0	10/1/2010
The NCCI edits preclude any payment for code **94010** when reported with code **94060** on the same date and by the same physician.			
90460 Immunization administration through 18 years of age, first or only component, with counseling by physician	**99392** Preventive medicine service, established patient age 1–4	1	1/1/2013
Unless modifier **25** (significant, separately identifiable E/M service) is appended to code **99392**, the charge associated with **99392** would be denied. Per *CPT*, immunization counseling is not included in preventive medicine E/M services. When both services are rendered on the same date, modifier **25** is appropriately appended to the code for the preventive medicine E/M service.			

Abbreviations: *CPT, Current Procedural Terminology*; E/M, evaluation and management; NCCI, National Correct Coding Initiative.

Medically Unlikely Edits

Medicare and Medicaid NCCI edits also include MUEs that place a limit on the number of units of service per code that will be allowed per date of service based on the number most likely to be billed in a single day by all health care professionals. Medically Unlikely Edits are intended to prevent payment for an inappropriate number or quantity of the same service.

An MUE for a Healthcare Common Procedure Coding System (HCPCS)/*Current Procedural Terminology* (*CPT®*) code is the maximum number of units of service, under most circumstances, allowable by the same provider for the same patient on the same date of service. Other health plans may also utilize unit of service edits. Ensure you know which MUE set a health plan is applying to your claims; the Medicaid MUEs are better associated with pediatric practice.

Medically Unlikely Edits are created based on

- Anatomical consideration
- Centers for Medicare & Medicaid Services policy
- Clinical CMS work group
- Clinical data
- Clinical society comment
- Code descriptor/*CPT* instruction
- Compounded drug policy

> ### Know Which Medically Unlikely Edits Plans Apply
>
> Ensure you know which Medically Unlikely Edit (MUE) set a health plan is applying to your claims. The Medicaid MUEs are better associated with pediatric practice.

- Drug discontinued
- Nature of analyte
- Nature of equipment
- Nature of service/procedure
- Oral medication; not payable
- Prescribing information
- Published contractor policy

Examples of Medically Unlikely Edits

The Medicaid MUE for initial hospital care code 99291 is 1 because this code describes only the initial 30 to 74 minutes of critical care on any date per *CPT* instruction. Additional time spent providing critical care on the same date is reported with code 99292 with 1 unit for each additional 30 minutes. The Medicaid MUE for 99292 is 8 units.

99291	Critical care, evaluation and management of the critically ill or critically injured patient; first 30-74 minutes
99292	Critical care, evaluation and management of the critically ill or critically injured patient; each additional 30 minutes

The Medicaid MUE for code 90460 is 9, reflecting the highest number of separate vaccine/toxoid products likely to be administered on a single date based on Advisory Committee on Immunization Practices recommendations.

90460	Immunization administration through 18 years of age via any route of administration, with counseling by physician or other qualified health care professional; first or only component of each vaccine or toxoid administered

Some, but not all, MUEs can be overridden by use of modifiers and/or separate claim lines.

- Medicaid MUEs are applied separately to each line of a claim. If the unit of service on a line exceeds the MUE value, the entire line is denied.
- If billed on separate lines with an appropriate modifier, all services may be paid.

Physicians shall not inconvenience beneficiaries nor increase risks to beneficiaries by performing services on different dates of service to avoid Medically Unlikely Edit or National Correct Coding Initiative procedure-to-procedure edits.

Example

> The mother, teacher, and maternal and paternal grandmothers each complete the Parents' Evaluation of Developmental Status screening form. The screenings are scored and interpreted. The pediatrician's claim includes 2 lines for these services.
>
> **96110** × 3 units (developmental screening with scoring and documentation)
>
> **96110 59** × 1 unit
>
> Medicaid MUEs place a per-claim line limit of 3 units of service for **96110** (developmental screening [eg, developmental milestone survey, speech and language delay screen], with scoring and documentation, per standardized instrument). When more than 3 units are clinically justified, the edit may be bypassed by reporting 3 units of service on one claim line and appending modifier **59** (distinct procedural service) to additional claim lines.
>
> Health plans may assign different reporting requirements for these services and, in addition, may have different upper limits on the number of units allowed.

Modifiers

Some code edits may be overridden by use of a modifier. A modifier indicator, **0** or **1**, advises whether use of a clinically justified modifier will result in override of the code pair edit.

> **0**: The code pair cannot be billed under any circumstances.
>
> **1**: An NCCI-associated modifier will override the edit.

- Certain modifiers can be used to override NCCI edits when the service or procedure is clinically justified, and they may be used only on the code pairs that are assigned the **1** indicator. (See modifiers in **Table 6-2**.)
  - > Medicaid NCCI-associated modifiers do not include
    - **22** (increased procedural services)
    - **76** (repeat procedure or service by same physician or other qualified health care professional)
    - **77** (repeat procedure or service by another physician or other qualified health care professional)
  - > Use of any of these modifiers does not bypass an NCCI code pair edit.

To append the appropriate modifier and override an edit, it is imperative that the conditions of that modifier are met.

Table 6-2. Modifiers That Can Be Used to Override National Correct Coding Initiative Edits		
24	Unrelated E/M service by the same physician or other QHP during a postoperative period	F6	Right hand, second digit
		F7	Right hand, third digit
25	Significant, separately identifiable E/M service by the same physician or other QHP on the same day of the procedure or other service	F8	Right hand, fourth digit
		F9	Right hand, fifth digit
		LC	Left circumflex, coronary artery
57	Decision for surgery	LD	Left anterior descending coronary artery
58	Staged or related procedure or service by the same physician or other QHP during the postoperative period	LM	Left main coronary artery
		LT	Left side
		RC	Right coronary artery
59	Distinct procedural service	RI	Ramus intermedius coronary artery
78	Unplanned return to the operating/ procedure room by the same physician or other QHP following initial procedure for a related procedure during the postoperative period	RT	Right side
		TA	Left foot, great toe
		T1	Left foot, second digit
		T2	Left foot, third digit
79	Unrelated procedure or service by the same physician or other QHP during the postoperative period	T3	Left foot, fourth digit
		T4	Left foot, fifth digit
		T5	Right foot, great toe
91	Repeat clinical diagnostic laboratory test	T6	Right foot, second digit
E1	Upper left, eyelid	T7	Right foot, third digit
E2	Lower left, eyelid	T8	Right foot, fourth digit
E3	Upper right, eyelid	T9	Right foot, fifth digit
E4	Lower right, eyelid	XE	Separate encounter (different operative session)
FA	Left hand, thumb		
F1	Left hand, second digit	XP	Separate practitioner
F2	Left hand, third digit	XS	Separate structure (site/organ)
F3	Left hand, fourth digit	XU	Unusual nonoverlapping service
F4	Left hand, fifth digit		
F5	Right hand, thumb		

Abbreviations: E/M, evaluation and management; QHP, qualified health care professional.

Example

> You provide and document an age- and gender- appropriate preventive E/M service and immunization administrations on the same date.

> The NCCI edits bundle the preventive E/M service codes with codes for immunization administration. However, it is appropriate to append modifier **25** (significant, separately identifiable E/M service) to the code for the preventive E/M service because this service is significantly beyond any preservice and post-service work of the immunization administration.

> ### Modifier 25 and 99211
>
> Most health plans will not allow payment for code **99211** (evaluation and management service not requiring the presence of a physician or other qualified health care professional [nursing visit]) on the same date as immunization administration. Modifier **25** will not override this edit.

Global Period Edits

Many codes for procedural services are valued to include certain preservice and post-service work. The period during which other services are considered inclusive to a procedure is the *global period*.

- Global periods and minor or major surgery are not defined in *CPT*.
- *CPT* directs that each procedure code represents a "surgical package" of service components. These include
  - > Evaluation and management services subsequent to the decision for surgery on the day before and/or day of surgery (including the history and physical examination)
  - > Local or topical anesthesia, including metacarpal, metatarsal, and/or digital block
  - > Immediate postoperative care
  - > Writing orders
  - > Evaluation of the patient in the recovery area
  - > Typical postoperative follow-up care
- The Medicare Physician Fee Schedule (MPFS) assigns global periods based on whether a procedure is minor or major.
  - > Most minor procedures are assigned a 0- or 10-day global period.
  - > Major procedures are assigned a 90-day global period.
  - > The day of surgery is day 0 (zero); the postoperative period begins the next day.
  - > Current Medicare global period assignments are available at www.cms.gov/apps/physician-fee-schedule/overview.aspx.

> What if the patient returns for an unrelated visit during a global period?
>
> Unrelated visits may be reported and are identified by addition of modifier **24** (unrelated E/M service by the same physician or other QHP during a postoperative period).

- Although other health plans can assign different global periods, most follow the MPFS. Be sure to obtain each plan's global period rules prior to accepting a contract requiring you to follow those rules.

Codes with global periods are identified by claims adjudication systems, which will then deny charges for services such as follow-up visits provided within the global period. As with other edits, modifiers may be used when clinically justified to override a global period edit.

Examples

A pediatric surgeon returns to the operating room to stop bleeding from an abdominal procedure performed earlier in the day.

The surgeon reports **35840 78** (exploration for postoperative hemorrhage, thrombosis, or infection; abdomen).

Modifier **78** is appended to code **35840** to indicate an unplanned return to the operating/procedure room by the same physician following an initial procedure for a related procedure during the postoperative period.

A patient has closed treatment of a shoulder dislocation with manipulation; 2 months later, the patient requires open treatment of a humeral shaft fracture.

The surgeon reports **24515 79** (open treatment of humeral shaft fracture with plate/screws, with or without cerclage).

Modifier **79** is appended to code **24515** to indicate an unrelated procedure was performed by the same physician or a physician of the same specialty and same group practice within the global period of a prior procedure.

Codes and Payment Policies

Many health plans publish payment policies that provide guidance on whether a service is covered under the plan and/or for what conditions a service may be covered. Never apply one health plan's policies to all your claims for services, as policies and payment vary by plan.

> **Applying Health Plan Policies**
>
> Never apply one health plan's policies to all your claims for services, as policies and payment vary by plan.

Examples of Health Plan Policies

- Visual function screening (**99172**) is included in the preventive medicine services and not separately payable.

- Visual acuity screening (**99173**) is separately payable for members younger than 22 years.

- Application of fluoride varnish by a primary care physician during an Early and Periodic Screening, Diagnostic, and Treatment visit must be billed using *CPT* code **99188** (application of topical fluoride varnish by a physician or other qualified health care professional) and *International Classification of Diseases, 10th Revision, Clinical Modification* code **Z29.3** (encounter for prophylactic fluoride administration).

Awareness and periodic monitoring of the policies of local and regional health plans helps pediatric practices know what services health plans cover and any related coding requirements.

Coding Keys

- **Medical necessity:** Typically, health plans will only pay for recommended preventive services and services that are medically necessary. That means they typically do not cover cosmetic procedures unless the procedure is also therapeutic or improves the function of a body part.

- **The importance of coding compliance:** Taking the time to learn about and support compliant coding and billing practices typically results in more accurate payment as well as the avoidance of risks associated with coding errors, including

  > Denied claims

  > Underpayment or overpayment that requires reconciliation with a payer and/or patient

  > Recoupment of amounts previously paid

  > Potential violations of fraud and abuse regulations and associated penalties

- **Code edits:** Code edits are one method for ensuring that benefits are paid only for medically necessary and/or preventive services covered by a health plan. They are used to automate the claims adjudication process. Edits allow electronic programs to either allow or deny charges for services based on each claim line.

- **National Correct Coding Initiative (NCCI) edits:** NCCI edits are sets of claim processing edits used by Medicare and Medicaid programs. They were developed to promote national correct coding methodologies and reduce improper coding that could lead to inappropriate payment in Medicare Part B claims. The NCCI has now expanded to be used by many private and government-funded health plans. There are 2 types of NCCI edits.

  > Procedure-to-procedure (PTP) edits prevent improper payment when incorrect code combinations are reported.

  > Medically Unlike Edits (MUEs) limit the number of units of service allowed on one date to help eliminate inaccurate payment caused by errors in the number of units reported.

- **Modifiers:** Some modifiers can override code edits. A modifier indicator (either **0** or **1**) denotes whether use of a clinically justified modifier will result in overriding the code edit.

  > **0**: The code pair cannot be billed under any circumstances.

  > **1**: An NCCI-associated modifier will override the edit.

- **Global period edits:** Many codes for procedural services are valued to include preservice and post-service work. The period during which other services are considered inclusive to a procedure is the *global period*.

Resources

American Academy of Pediatrics

- Coding Hotline (www.aap.org/en-us/Pages/cu/Coding-Hotline-Request.aspx)
- Coding Webinars (www.aap.org/en-us/professional-resources/practice-transformation/getting-paid/Coding-at-the-AAP/Pages/AAP-Coding-Webinars.aspx)
- *AAP Pediatric Coding Newsletter*™ (http://coding.aap.org)
- Coding Calculator (www.aap.org/en-us/professional-resources/practice-transformation/getting-paid/Coding-at-the-AAP/Pages/Coding-Calculator.aspx)

Payment/Denial Advocacy

- Payer Advocacy Templates for Appeal Letters (www.aap.org/en-us/professional-resources/practice-transformation/getting-paid/Pages/Private-Payer-Advocacy-Templates-for-Appeal-Letters.aspx)
- Payer Advocacy: Letters to Carriers (www.aap.org/en-us/professional-resources/practice-transformation/getting-paid/Pages/Private-Payer-Advocacy-Letters-to-Carriers.aspx)
- AAP Pediatric Councils (www.aap.org/en-us/professional-resources/practice-transformation/getting-paid/Pages/aap-pediatric-councils.aspx)
- Oops We've Overpaid You: How to Respond to Payer Audits (https://www.aap.org/en-us/professional-resources/practice-transformation/getting-paid/pages/Oops-We-Overpaid-You-How-to-Respond-to-Payer-Audits.aspx)
- Reporting Inappropriate Denials: Hassle Factor Form (www.aap.org/en-us/professional-resources/practice-transformation/getting-paid/Pages/Hassle-Factor-Form-Concerns-with-Payers.aspx)

Documentation

- Program Integrity: Documentation Matters Toolkit (www.cms.gov/Medicare-Medicaid-Coordination/Fraud-Prevention/Medicaid-Integrity-Education/documentation-matters.html)
- National Committee for Quality Assurance (www.ncqa.org)

Immunization and Vaccines

- American Medical Association Category I vaccine codes (www.ama-assn.org/practice-management/cpt/category-i-vaccine-codes)
- Centers for Disease Control and Prevention (CDC) Vaccines for Children program (www.cdc.gov/vaccines/programs/vfc/index.html)
- Coding at the AAP (www.aap.org/en-us/professional-resources/practice-transformation/getting-paid/Coding-at-the-AAP/Pages/Vaccine-Coding.aspx)
  - > Vaccine Counseling and Preventive Care Visits
  - > Influenza Vaccines: Coding for the Current Season
  - > Vaccine Coding Table

> When Is It Appropriate to Report an E/M Service During Immunization Administration?
> FAQ—Pediatric Immunization Administration Codes
> CDC Vaccine Price List
> New Versus Established Patient Status After Vaccine Only Encounter

- American Academy of Pediatrics *Pediatric Vaccines: Coding Quick Reference Card* (https://shop.aap.org)

Legal Advice

- American Health Lawyers Association (www.healthlawyers.org)
- Centers for Medicare & Medicaid Services Medicare global period assignments (www.cms.gov/apps/physician-fee-schedule/overview.aspx)
- National Correct Coding Initiative edits (www.cms.gov/NationalCorrectCodInitEd/NCCIEP/list.asp)

Payer Audits

- Payer Contract Negotiations and Payment Resources (www.aap.org/en-us/professional-resources/practice-transformation/getting-paid/Pages/payer-contract-negotiations-and-payment-resources.aspx; access code AAPCFP25)
- Medicaid Recovery Audit Contractor program (https://hms.com/medicaid-recovery-audit-contractor)

Surgery

- Centers for Medicare & Medicaid Services–designated global periods, Medicare Resource-Based Relative Value Scale Physician Fee Schedule (www.cms.gov/Medicare/Medicare-Fee-for-Service-Payment/PhysicianFeeSched/PFS-Relative-Value-Files.html; see column O)

Current Procedural Terminology

- American Academy of Pediatrics *Coding for Pediatrics* (www.aap.org/cfp)
- American Medical Association *CPT* general information (www.ama-assn.org/practice-management/cpt-current-procedural-terminology)

International Classification of Diseases, 10th Revision, Clinical Modification Code Files and Guidelines

- American Academy of Pediatrics *Pediatric ICD-10-CM: A Manual for Provider-Based Coding* (https://shop.aap.org)
- National Center for Health Statistics *ICD-10-CM* (www.cdc.gov/nchs/icd/icd10cm.htm)

Coding Challenge

(Answers may be found in Appendix A.)

1. Health care interventions that are medically necessary are which of the following?

   a. Evidence based, evidence informed, or based on consensus advisory opinion

   b. Any interventions that can be assigned a procedure code

   c. Only those that are covered by individual health plan benefits

   d. Any intervention that a patient/caregiver requests

2. A code pair is listed in the procedure-to-procedure National Correct Coding Initiative (NCCI) edits with a modifier indicator of **0** (zero). What does the modifier indicator mean?

   a. The code pair is not subject to NCCI edits.

   b. A health plan will not pay for either service.

   c. The code pair edit cannot be overridden by use of a modifier.

   d. You should append a modifier to the code in the second column.

3. Which of the following is not included in the surgical package as defined by *Current Procedural Terminology*?

   a. A return to the operating room for treatment of a surgical complication

   b. Writing orders

   c. Evaluation of the patient in the recovery area

   d. Local anesthesia

4. How long are the typical global periods of services?

   a. 0, 10, or 60 days following the service

   b. 0, 10, or 90 days, including the date of the service

   c. 0, 10, or 90 days following the date of the service

   d. All pediatric services include a 90-day global period.

Appendix A

Coding Challenge Answer Key

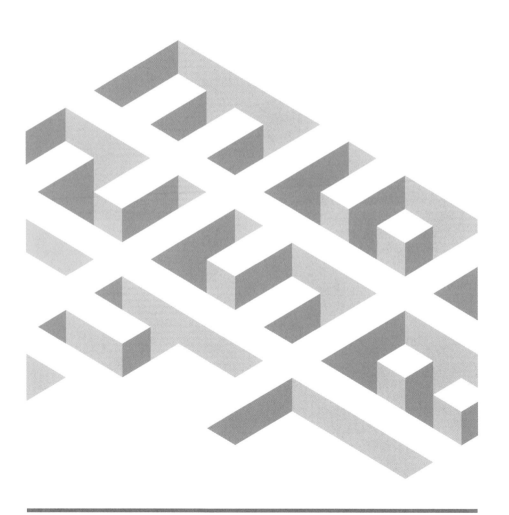

Chapter 1

1. How many Health Insurance Portability and Accountability Act of 1996 (HIPAA)-designated code sets can be used in reporting pediatric professional services?

    a. 2

    b. 3

    c. 4

    d. 5

    Answer: c. The code sets are *International Classification of Diseases, 10th Revision, Clinical Modification (ICD-10-CM)*; *Current Procedural Terminology (CPT®)*; Healthcare Common Procedure Coding System (HCPCS); and National Drug Code (NDC).

2. The rationale for ordering diagnostic and other ancillary services should be what?

    a. Included on the claim form

    b. Documented

    c. Easily inferred

    d. b and c

    Answer: d. If not documented, the rationale for ordering diagnostic and other ancillary services should be easily inferred.

3. Which of the following is mandated by HIPAA?

    a. Everyone must have health insurance.

    b. Codes for reporting medical services

    c. Specific claim forms (electronic and paper)

    d. b and c

    Answer: d. HIPAA mandates specific claim forms (electronic and paper) and codes for reporting medical services.

4. Who certifies the correctness of the information on each claim submitted for payment?

    a. The billing staff who prepare claims for submission

    b. The pediatrician or other provider of service

    c. The patient

    d. A practice manager or administrator

    Answer: b. The individual who is listed as the provider of service attests to the accuracy of information submitted on each claim.

Chapter 2

1. What does *ICD* stand for?

   a. *International Classification of Death*

   b. *International Classification of Diseases*

   c. *Independent Categorization of Disease*

   d. *Independent Classification of Diseases*

   Answer: b. *ICD* stands for *International Classification of Diseases*.

2. How many characters are placed to the left of the decimal point in an *International Classification of Diseases, 10th Revision, Clinical Modification (ICD-10-CM)* code?

   a. 7

   b. 3

   c. Up to 4

   d. 2

   Answer: b. Three characters are placed to the left of the decimal. Codes appear in the following pattern: **XXX.XXXX**.

3. What letter is used to fill the fourth through sixth characters when necessary to support addition of a seventh character?

   a. X

   b. O

   c. None; a dash (-) is used.

   d. None; the seventh character is inserted in place of the fourth through sixth characters.

   Answer: a. An **X** is used to complete the fourth through sixth characters when a seventh character is required to complete a code.

4. What claim item on the 1500 claim form is used to link diagnosis pointers to procedure codes?

   a. Item 21

   b. Item 24D

   c. Item 24E

   d. Item 24B

   Answer: c. Item 24E is the diagnosis pointer that carries the letter of each diagnosis code entered into the fields in item 21 to the services lines in item 24.

Chapter 3

1. In which *Current Procedural Terminology* (*CPT*) appendix will you find a listing of modifiers?

    a. Appendix A

    b. Appendix B

    c. Appendix M

    d. Appendix X

    Answer: a. Appendix A lists each modifier and its description.

2. Which of the following is not a criterion for Category I creation in *CPT*?

    a. Paid by many health plans

    b. Performed by most health care professionals, including pediatricians, in the United States

    c. Performed at a frequency consistent with clinical indications and current medical practice

    d. The efficacy of the service is supported in medical literature.

    Answer: a. Answers b, c, and d are the criteria for a new *CPT* Category I code. Payment by health plans is not a criterion for code assignment. Also, code assignment does not guarantee payment.

3. A code preceded by a plus sign (+) is

    a. A new code

    b. An add-on code

    c. A code for new or emerging technology

    d. A service that may be provided via telemedicine

    Answer: b. The plus sign (+) symbolizes an add-on code that is always reported in conjunction with another code.

4. When selecting a *CPT* code, which of the following is true?

    a. Codes should be selected from the alphabetical index alone.

    b. A code that approximates the service provided is sufficient.

    c. Never select an unlisted procedure code.

    d. Use the guidelines and instructions in the numerical listing to guide code selection.

    Answer: d. Code selection should always include review of the numerical listing to verify that the code descriptor is appropriate to the service provided and that the service is reported in compliance with the guidelines and instructions applicable to the code.

Chapter 4

1. True or false? Healthcare Common Procedure Coding System (HCPCS) codes are composed of 5 numerical characters.

    a. True

    b. False

    Answer: b. False. HCPCS codes are alphanumeric with 1 letter followed by 4 numbers.

2. What information is included in the HCPCS Table of Drugs?

    a. Brand names of medications

    b. Generic names of medications

    c. Method of administration

    d. All of the above

    Answer: d. In addition to brand and generic names, the table includes the method of administration and the amount of the drug that equals 1 unit of service.

3. Which of the following indicates the laterality of a procedure or service?

    a. Modifier **XE**

    b. Modifier **QW**

    c. HCPCS code

    d. Modifier **LT** or **RT**

    Answer: d. Modifiers LT (left) and RT (right) may be appended to the code for a procedure or service to indicate laterality.

4. How often are HCPCS code updates implemented?

    a. Annually, January 1

    b. Each January 1, with quarterly updates for temporary codes

    c. October 1

    d. As needed throughout the year

    Answer: b. HCPCS codes are updated annually on January 1. However, the Centers for Medicare & Medicaid Services may add temporary codes quarterly.

Chapter 5

1. Correctly assigning and linking diagnosis codes to services and supplies on a claim provides a health plan with what information?

    a. The reason that each service or supply was clinically indicated

    b. What services were provided

    c. Alterations or special circumstances in how a service was provided

    d. All of the above

    Answer: d. Correctly assigned and linked codes and modifiers provide a health plan with the reasons for services and supplies, what services and supplies were provided, and any alterations or special circumstances related to services provided.

2. True or false? You must assign only one diagnosis per claim line.

    a. True

    b. False

    Answer: b. False. Up to 4 diagnosis codes may be linked to each service line on a claim.

3. What do you call the amount you must adjust off your charge because of your contractual agreement with the health plan?

    a. Deductible

    b. Patient balance

    c. Contractual adjustment

    d. Modifier

    Answer: c. A *contractual adjustment* is the amount you must adjust off your charge because of your contractual agreement with the health plan.

4. What is a *clean claim*?

    a. A claim with only one service line

    b. A claim containing all information necessary for the health plan to determine benefit payments

    c. A claim that is filed on the same date the service was provided

    d. A claim that contains up to 6 service lines

    Answer: b. Clean claims contain all information necessary for the health plan to determine benefit payments and are subject to prompt payment regulations in most states.

Chapter 6

1. Health care interventions that are medically necessary are which of the following?

    a. Evidence based, evidence informed, or based on consensus advisory opinion

    b. Any interventions that can be assigned a procedure code

    c. Only those that are covered by individual health plan benefits

    d. Any intervention that a patient/caregiver requests

    Answer: a. The American Academy of Pediatrics (AAP) defines *medical necessity* as health care interventions that are evidence based, evidence informed, or based on consensus advisory opinion and are recommended by recognized health care professionals, such as the AAP, to promote optimal growth and development in a child and to prevent, detect, diagnose, treat, ameliorate, or palliate the effects of physical, genetic, congenital, developmental, behavioral, or mental conditions, injuries, or disabilities.

2. A code pair is listed in the procedure-to-procedure National Correct Coding Initiative (NCCI) edits with a modifier indicator of **0** (zero). What does the modifier indicator mean?

    a. The code pair is not subject to NCCI edits.

    b. A health plan will not pay for either service.

    c. The code pair edit cannot be overridden by use of a modifier.

    d. You should append a modifier to the code in the second column.

    Answer: c. Modifier indicator 0 means no modifier will override the edits. Modifier indicator 1 means a modifier may override the edits when clinically justified.

3. Which of the following is not included in the surgical package as defined by *Current Procedural Terminology*?

    a. A return to the operating room for treatment of a surgical complication

    b. Writing orders

    c. Evaluation of the patient in the recovery area

    d. Local anesthesia

    Answer: a. *Current Procedural Terminology* does not include treatment of surgical complications in the surgical package.

4. How long are the typical global periods of services?

    a. 0, 10, or 60 days following the service

    b. 0, 10, or 90 days, including the date of the service

    c. 0, 10, or 90 days following the date of the service

    d. All pediatric services include a 90-day global period.

    Answer: c. Global periods of 0, 10, or 90 days are used by Medicare and most other payers.

Appendix B

Glossary of Common Coding Acronyms

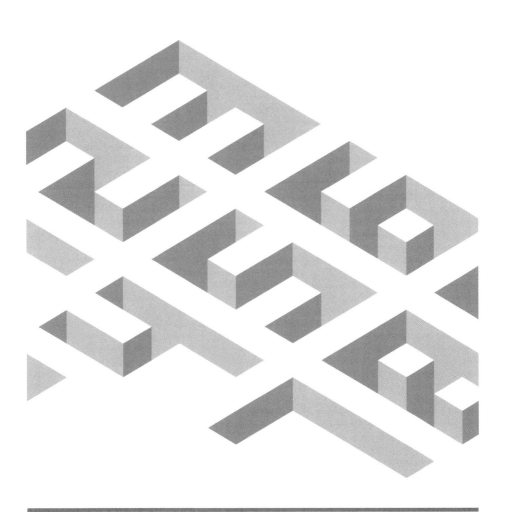

AAP	American Academy of Pediatrics
AHA	American Hospital Association
AMA	American Medical Association
ASC	ambulatory surgery center
CF	conversion factor
CLIA	Clinical Laboratory Improvement Amendments
CMS	Centers for Medicare & Medicaid Services
COCN	Committee on Coding and Nomenclature
CPT®	*Current Procedural Terminology*®
EHR	electronic health record
E/M	evaluation and management
EPSDT	Early and Periodic Screening, Diagnostic, and Treatment
FDA	US Food and Drug Administration
GPCI	geographic practice cost index
HCPCS	Healthcare Common Procedure Coding System
HIPAA	Health Insurance Portability and Accountability Act of 1996
ICD-10-CM	*International Classification of Diseases, 10th Revision, Clinical Modification*
MPFS	Medicare Physician Fee Schedule
MUE	Medically Unlikely Edit
NCCI	National Correct Coding Initiative
NDC	National Drug Code
NEC	Not elsewhere classifiable. When used in the *ICD-10-CM* alphabetic index, NEC indicates the index is pointing to an "other specified" code in the tabular list. Other specified codes are used when a specific code is not available for a condition.
NOC	Not otherwise classified
NOS	Not otherwise specified. This abbreviation is the equivalent of unspecified.
NUCC	National Uniform Claim Committee
OPPS	Outpatient Prospective Payment System
PCP	primary care professional
PTP	procedure-to-procedure (code edits)
QHP	qualified health care professional (eg, advanced practice registered nurse, physician assistant)
RVU	relative value unit

Appendix C

History of Medical Payment

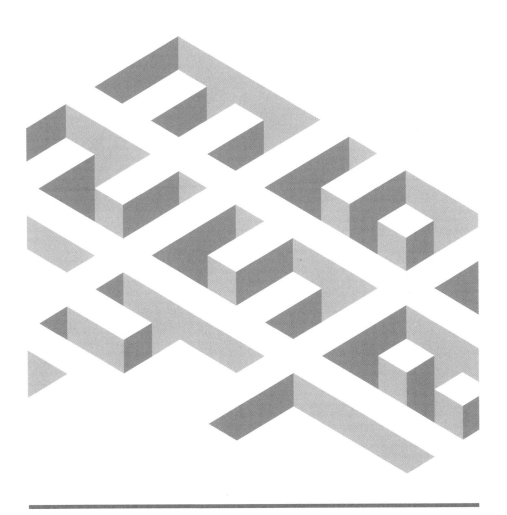

Before health insurance was common, patients paid cash or other items or services of value (eg, chickens, plumbing) directly to pediatricians at the time of service. This slowly changed over time until 1965, when President Lyndon B. Johnson signed Medicare and Medicaid into law. Soon after, it became more common for physicians to sign contracts to participate in government health programs and the provider networks of health plans. Getting paid got more complicated.

It became necessary for the physician to bill the health plan rather than or prior to billing the patient or caregiver. Health plans only paid for certain services (eg, care for acute or chronic physical illness) and excluded others (eg, preventive services); so, a detailed statement of charges with a reason or diagnosis for each service provided was required. These detailed statements or claims were not standardized and often were handwritten or typed. The lack of standardized terminology and format caused significant delays and errors in claim processing.

Diagnosis Coding

Coding resulted from the need to classify the causes of mortality and, later, morbidity. In the late 1800s, countries began collaborating to develop standardized nomenclatures and classifications of mortality. Disease classification was added over time (**Figure C-1**).

- The current World Health Organization (WHO) *International Classification of Diseases (ICD)* can trace its origins to the International Causes of Death (Bertillon Classification) in 1893. Decennial revisions were introduced in 1900. This process was interrupted by World War II.

- The United States first combined a morbidity and mortality classification system in 1910 with the publication of *International Classification of Causes of Sickness and Death*.

- The newly formed WHO took over control of *ICD* with the publication of *ICD-6* in 1948.

- The first US modification of *ICD* was published by the US Public Health Service in 1968.

- Today the *International Classification of Diseases, 10th Revision (ICD-10)* is used in more than 100 countries, including the United States.

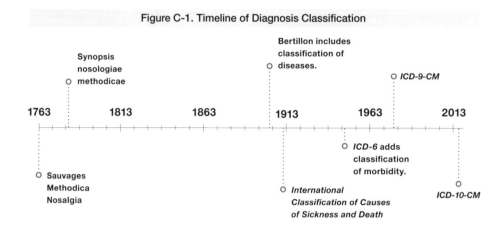

Figure C-1. Timeline of Diagnosis Classification

Current Procedural Terminology® Codes

While *Current Procedural Terminology (CPT)* is part of the Healthcare Common Procedure Coding System (HCPCS) code set now, it was not always so. Table C-1 illustrates the timeline of *CPT* development and adoption as a standard code set.

CPT was developed in its initial form in 1966, long before the Level II HCPCS codes. The initial *CPT* focused mainly on surgical services and has grown substantially since that time. The American Medical Association began licensing the *CPT* code set as HCPCS Level I codes to the Health Care Finance Administration (now the Centers for Medicare & Medicaid Services) in 1983. Prior to that time, *CPT* codes were not required on Medicare and Medicaid claims. In 1996, the Health Insurance Portability and Accountability Act regulations formally required use of *CPT* and HCPCS Level II Codes by all covered entities (most physicians and health plans).

Table C-1. History of *Current Procedural Terminology*				
1966	1976	1977	1983-1986	2000
1st Edition *CPT*	3rd Edition *CPT*	4th Edition *CPT*	CPT/HCPCS	HIPAA
The American Medical Association publishes first 4-digit *CPT* codes primarily for surgical procedures.	*CPT* is expanded to 5 digits and includes more diagnostic and therapeutic procedures.	System of periodic updating introduced to *CPT* (now *CPT* Editorial Panel and Advisory Committee).	*CPT* became a part of the HCPCS code set used by Medicare and Medicaid. *CPT* mandated for outpatient hospital surgical procedures reported to Medicare/Medicaid.	*CPT* becomes a standard code set used by all covered entities under HIPAA.

Abbreviations: CPT, *Current Procedural Terminology;* HCPCS, Healthcare Common Procedure Coding System; HIPAA, Health Insurance Portability and Accountability Act of 1996.

Healthcare Common Procedure Coding System Codes

HCPCS codes were initially developed between 1977 and 1983 in an effort to bring uniformity to coding for professional services. There were multiple coding systems in use across Medicare contractors, Medicaid plans, and private payers at the time. **Table C-2** shows key changes from establishment to standardization of the HCPCS code set.

Table C-2. Timeline of Healthcare Common Procedure Coding System History			
1977	**1983**	**2000**	**December 31, 2003**
HCFA Charged to Establish Code Set	**HCPCS Required for Medicare**	**HCPCS Required Under HIPAA**	**HCPCS Level III Retired**
HCFA charged with establishing or adopting a uniform code set for physician services	In 1983, HCFA (now CMS) required all Medicare contractors to use HCPCS codes in claims adjudication.	HCPCS becomes a standard code set used by all covered entities under HIPAA.	As required under HIPAA, Level III HCPCS codes (created and used by local payers) were no longer HIPAA compliant.

Abbreviations: CMS, Centers for Medicare & Medicaid Services; HCFA, Health Care Finance Administration; HCPCS, Healthcare Common Procedure Coding System; HIPAA, Health Insurance Portability and Accountability Act of 1996.

Appendix D

Certificate of Completion

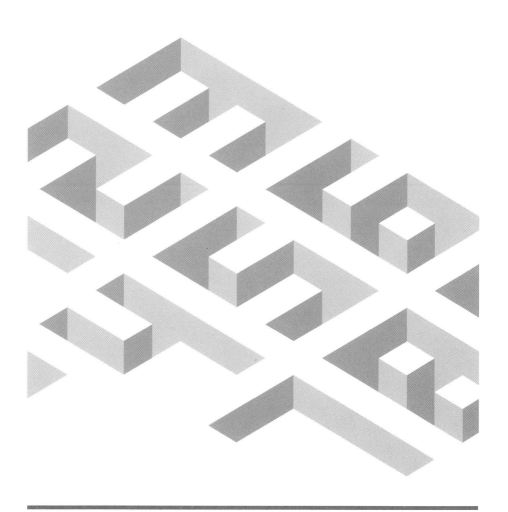

To further enhance your coding knowledge and obtain proof of your understanding of pediatric coding basics, an online quiz is available for you to complete. Upon successful completion of the quiz, you will obtain a Certificate of Completion from the American Academy of Pediatrics. To obtain this quiz please go to www.aap.org/PCBcertificate and access the online quiz.

Note: This quiz is not for official credit from any credentialing society.

Index

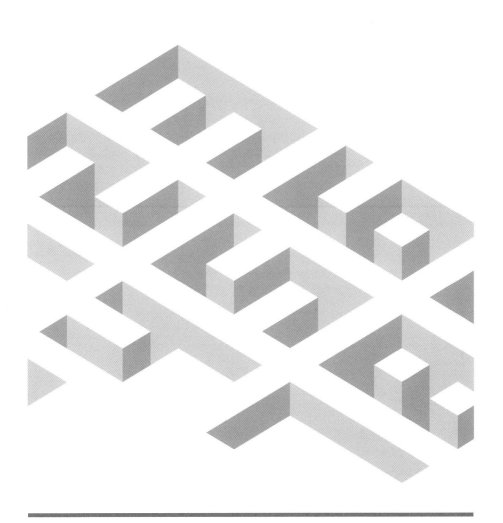

A

B

C

R

S

T

U

V

W

AAP Pediatric Coding Newsletter™

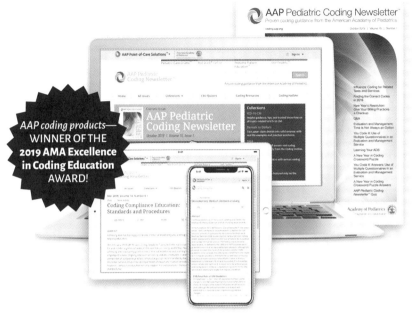

This print and online monthly publication brings you proven coding strategies, tips, and techniques you won't see in any other periodical. How-to help with your toughest coding challenges ensures that you get paid for all your work. The newsletter also features guidance and regular contributions from the AAP Committee on Coding and Nomenclature Editorial Advisory Board.

Issue after issue, *AAP Pediatric Coding* Newsletter gives the know-how needed to

- Reduce payment delays and claim denials.
- Increase diagnosis coding accuracy.
- Limit costly re-billing and appeals.
- Avoid payment shortfalls caused by down-coding.

SUBSCRIBE TODAY!

Visit **shop.aap.org/coding** or call toll-free **888-227-1770**

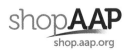

shop**AAP**
shop.aap.org

American Academy of Pediatrics
DEDICATED TO THE HEALTH OF ALL CHILDREN®